NONINVASIVE VENTILATION IN MEDICINE - RECENT UPDATES

Edited by **Mayank Vats**

Noninvasive Ventilation in Medicine - Recent Updates
http://dx.doi.org/10.5772/intechopen.68299
Edited by Mayank Vats

Contributors

Omid Fathi, Amy Schlegel, Edward Shepherd, Michalis Agrafiotis, Konstantina Nikolaou, Demetra Siopi, Diamantis Chloros, Jyothi Inampudi, Renuka Prasad Kowtha, Vijayakumar Thangavel Mahalingam, Rajalakshmi Rajagopalan, Ilango Kaliappan, R.C.Satish Kumar, Ramphanindra Talatam, Lavinia Davidescu, Diana Manolescu, Ruxandra Ulmeanu, Cristian Oancea, Elisabete Aramendi, Andoni Elola, Erik Alonso, Unai Irusta, Mayank Gyan Vats

First published in London, United Kingdom, 2019 by IntechOpen
IntechOpen is the global imprint of INTECHOPEN LIMITED, registered in England and Wales, registration number: 11086078, The Shard, 25th floor, 32 London Bridge Street
London, SE19SG – United Kingdom
Printed in Croatia

British Library Cataloguing-in-Publication Data
A catalogue record for this book is available from the British Library

Additional hard copies can be obtained from orders@intechopen.com

Noninvasive Ventilation in Medicine - Recent Updates, Edited by Mayank Vats
p. cm.
Print ISBN 978-1-78985-289-9
Online ISBN 978-1-78985-290-5

For EU product safety concerns:
IN TECH d.o.o., Prolaz Marije Krucifikse Kozulić 3, 51000 Rijeka, Croatia, info@intechopen.com or visit our website at intechopen.com.

Meet the editor

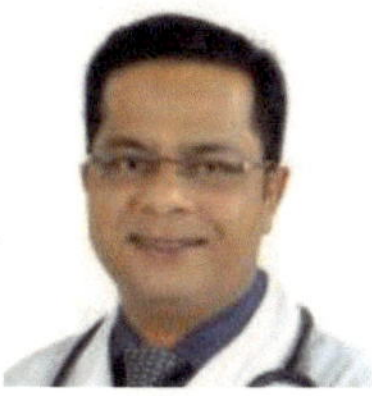

Dr Mayank Vats is a Senior Specialist, Interventional Pulmonologist, Pulmonologist, Intensivist, and Sleep Physician at Rashid Hospital and Dubai Hospital and developed the interventional pulmonology department in Rashid Hospital. Before coming to the United Arab Emirates, he was a consultant in Respiratory Medicine, Critical Care Medicine, and Sleep Medicine at Escorts Heart Institute and Apollo Hospital, New Delhi India, a tertiary level of care hospital in India. Dr Vats's interest is to utilize his professional knowledge and interpersonal skills in order to provide the highest degree of patient care and satisfaction. Having worked in a busy tertiary level teaching hospital and specialty corporate hospitals as a consultant, he has been exposed to the complete spectrum of respiratory, critical care and sleep medicine.

Contents

Preface

With the widespread pandemic of COPD , obesity, OSA, and cardiovascular diseases, noninvasive ventilation (NIV) has become a common and standard modality of care for such patients and these patients/diseases are the most common indications for NIV use as well as their role in other diseases such as neuromuscular disease and patients of tracheostomy and hypoxic respiratory failure as a bridge to avoid intubation pending the resolution of the primary disease and consequent hypoxia. NIV is a very simple and very important machine for the ICU physicians, anesthetists, pulmonologists, and many other specialties. Obtaining complete knowledge of how to operate and fine-tune the NIV is not difficult as there are hundreds of resources including websites, CMEs, conferences, and workshops available. The most important component of the NIV application in clinical practice is to gain expertise and experience in applying the technique and acquiring problem-solving skills.

A vast amount has been written about NIV, including books and guidelines hence we thought to produce a book called "Noninvasive Ventilation in Medicine - Recent Updates" to cover the untouched components of such this machine. In this book, we tried to include advances in the NIV and the how NIV could be used in synchrony with the mechanical ventilator including a weaning stage. The clinical scope of NIV is changing day-to-day and its rapidly emerging and constantly changing field includes many more indications of utilization of NIV. The current book contains a rich extract from the masters in the NIV field who have vast experience of NIV in areas other than conventional indications and would like to share their experience with all of the readers. Various challenges in NIV patient care include noncompliance, confused, hypercapnic patient or small children coping with a mask, avoiding interface leaks, and balancing ventilatory needs with patient tolerance.

We very much hope this book will help to broaden the scope of the NIV in clinical practice and will help readers to gain more insight and practical advice in NIV. I am extremely grateful to all the contributors and reviewers, and to IntechOpen for giving me the opportunity to prepare this book. Heartfelt thanks go to the publisher team (Ms Ana Panther, Ms Iva Lipovic, and others) for their great untiring support and enthusiasm. We are very much hopeful that this book "Noninvasive Ventilation in Medicine - Recent Updates" will help the target audience, pulmonary, internal medicine, sleep physicians gain a better understanding of disease and improved patient care.

I would like to extend my thanks to my parents (Dr Gian Chand Sharma and Mrs Kamla Vats) for their blessings, my family (wife Dr Deepa Vats, daughters Spraha and Aadhya) for their continuous support and IntechOpen publishing team for their great support and enthusiasm.

Dr Mayank Vats
MBBS, MD, DNB, FNB, MRCP, EDRM, FRCP, FACP, FCCP, MBA
Interventional Pulmonologist
Intensivist and Sleep Physician
Rashid Hospital
Dubai, United Arab Emirates

Chapter 1

Introductory: Non Invasive Ventilation in Medicine

Mayank Vats

Additional information is available at the end of the chapter

http://dx.doi.org/10.5772/intechopen.82663

1. Introduction

With the worldwide increasing use of noninvasive ventilation (NIV) and many updated evidences coming under the application of NIV in neuromuscular disease, neonates, and open circuit mouthpiece ventilation apart from the documented success of NIV in OSA, COPD, type 2 respiratory failure and pulmonary edema, it is the time to get more knowledge about its application for various chronic respiratory diseases such as interstitial lung disease and non-respiratory disease characterized by type 1 or type 2 respiratory failure in due course of time, and it is also important to know the potential application of NIV in children and neonates and as a mode for weaning from the mechanical ventilation, NIV is a rapidly changing field; hence, it is very important in clinical practice to have expertise in applying the technique and acquiring problem-solving skills of NIV.

If we go back to history, initially, negative pressure ventilators were invented primarily to tide over the ventilatory crisis of polio epidemic (epidemics of poliomyelitis), which had begun in the First World War and swept across Europe and the USA in the 1930s–1950s. They were of different types including cuirass ventilator, chest bellow, iron lung, tank ventilators, and many more but the main drawback with all these was that they were large, heavy, and cumbersome to operate and handle and were primarily used for the neuromuscular disease. Practical limitations were compounded by the huge outbreak of polio in Denmark in 1952, which was associated with a very high prevalence of cases with bulbar weakness. Not only an insufficient number of iron lungs were available, but these were also inadequate in caring for patients with bulbar problems—mortality rose to 90% and the only solution was invasive positive-pressure ventilation via a tracheostomy. This switch to positive pressure continued heralding the development of modern ICU. Later on, positive-pressure ventilators were developed with endotracheal intubation, which is a must for the application of these ventilators. From 1980 onward, positive pressure was applied through the face mask and found to be really effective for patients with COPD and obstructive sleep apnea, and it heralded the era of NIV globally. There was a brief resurgence of NIV in 1980s, but mainly to care for those with chronic ventilatory failure.

Long-term chronic use of NIV began to spur to ventilatory progress during 1980s. This was related to better understanding of the sleep physiology and the discovery of OSA and beneficial effects of CPAP. The original CPAP machines were very large, but newer machines are smaller, compact, and portable. Importantly, mask design and comfort has also improved, leading to success of NIV application. NIV is now one of the most evidence-based areas of respiratory medicine. NIV reduces mortality and morbidity in acute exacerbations of COPD, and this improved outcome in Duchenne muscle dystrophy and other neuromuscular diseases, OSA, in acute hypoxemic respiratory failure secondary to pulmonary edema and weaning from mechanical ventilation including high-risk patients for weaning. An additional major change in the past 30–40 years has been the increasing indications for long-term, chronic NIV and, of course, long-term application of CPAP in OSA.

For patients with a range of causes of ventilatory failure, the natural history progresses from normal breathing to a gradual loss in lung volumes and then, initially, changes in blood gases are seen at night due to hypoventilation, and if that is not addressed, ultimately, progress to daytime respiratory failure, cardiac decompensation, and premature death. In Duchenne muscular dystrophy and other neuromuscular diseases, once a patient starts developing high carbon dioxide level during the daytime and or night time, suggestive of ventilatory muscles fatigue and carries a dismal prognosis if the Home NIV support is not provided earliest possible. In COPD, recent trials have shown NIV may be beneficial in stable hypercapnic patients. NIV has been extended to the pediatric age range, with the feasibility of using NIV to control nocturnal hypoventilation in children initially being demonstrated predominantly in neuromuscular conditions. Many of these children now survive to adolescence or adulthood, as shown in the section entitled "Chronic NIV in hereditary neuromuscular disorders."

There is also growing interest in NIV in cardiology. There is no doubt that patients with heart disease and OSA benefit from treatment of the OSA. By contrast, Cheyne-Stokes respiration is a form of central sleep apnea in patients with chronic heart failure. Recent work shows that around half of patients with mild heart failure have sleep disordered breathing too. CPAP can be used to treat OSA, but it does not work in central sleep apnea or Cheyne-Stokes respiration. NIV is now being used in some situations to palliate symptoms without the aim of prolonging survival. Here, goals such as reduction in dyspnea and control of symptoms of nocturnal hypoventilation should be set preemptively so that if these are not met, NIV can be discontinued and palliative efforts are directed elsewhere. NIV combined with cough assist devices can also be used to manage severely ill type 1 spinal muscular atrophy infants with the aim of discharging the patient to their home and managing breathlessness.

2. Implementation of NIV in clinical practice

There is evidence that patients who would benefit from NIV are not receiving it even for gold standard indications, such as acute hypercapnic COPD, mainly because the medical team does

http://dx.doi.org/10.5772/intechopen.82663

not feel comfortable to start NIV; in such case, they must take MICU or pulmonary medicine doctor's opinion for the NIV in COPD and they must try to emphasize the use of NIV to the patients to improve quality of life and to reduce morbidity and mortality in not only COPD but also in all well-established indications for NIV use in various respiratory diseases. Pulmonary and MICU doctors are at forefront to recommend the use of NIV in established and potential indications to improve quality of life and survival.

Author details

Mayank Vats

Address all correspondence to: mvatsonline@gmail.com

Interventional Pulmonologist, Pulmonologist, Intensivist and Sleep Physician at Rashid Hospital and Dubai hospital, Dubai, UAE

Chapter 2

Obstructive Sleep Apnea: A Pathophysiology and Pharmacotherapy Approach

I Jyothi, K Renuka Prasad, R Rajalakshmi,
RC Satish Kumar, Talatam Ramphanindra,
TM Vijayakumar and Ilango Kaliappan

Additional information is available at the end of the chapter

http://dx.doi.org/10.5772/intechopen.77981

Abstract

Obstructive sleep apnea (OSA) is a common sleep disorder characterized by complete cessation of upper airflow during sleep, leading to repetitive episodes of desaturations and arousals. The symptoms include excessive daytime somnolence and are associated with a significant cardiovascular morbidity and mortality. The prevalence of OSA is higher in men with an approximate rate of 14 and 5% in women respectively. Typical risk factors for obstructive sleep apnea in the normal adult population are obesity, aging, gender, menopause, ethnicity, genetical predisposition, craniofacial anatomy, smoking, alcohol consumption and some other factors such as REM sleep, surface tension, and impaired sensory processing. Several screening questionnaires can be performed in outpatient settings to identify the patient symptoms. Polysomnography is considered as the gold standard for diagnosis of OSA. Different surgical treatments and devices are readily available for an effective management of this disease. Proper diagnosis and treatment improves not only the quality of life but also relatively decreases patient morbidity and mortality. A multifaceted approach is necessary for an accurate management of the OSA.

Keywords: obstructive sleep apnea, excessive daytime somnolence, obesity, polysomnography, quality of life

1. Introduction

The first clear modern description of obstructive sleep apnea (OSA) was given by Burwell in 1956 in the publication entitled, "Extreme Obesity Associated with Alveolar Hypoventilation:

A Pickwickian Syndrome." The name came from Charles Dickens' The Posthumous Papers of the Pickwick Club (1837). It is unclear if the patient named Joe with overweight exhibited symptoms of OSA, and it took another decade before Gastaut and colleagues in 1966 recognized OSA in obese patients and noted these nocturnal disturbances to possibly be linked to their daytime somnolence [1].

Obstructive sleep apnea (OSA) is a potentially serious and life-threatening disorder affecting millions of people around the world. It is a sleep-related respiratory condition, characterized by the complete or partial collapse of breathing because of a narrowing or closure of the upper airway during sleep, resulting in intermittent cessations of breathing (apneas) or reductions in airflow (hypopneas) despite ongoing respiratory effort [2]. The symptoms include excessive daytime sleepiness, Mood changes, Fragmented sleep, as well as the decreased health-related quality of life. Patients often complain of snoring, Gasping or choking, frequent nocturnal awakenings, early morning headaches, poor concentration and coordination, anxiety, irritability, and insomnia, yet many patients are unaware of these symptoms and disease onset is insidious [3, 4]. The underlying mechanism of OSA is still under investigation, but it is precisely multifaceted.

The economic burden of OSA is substantial due to its high prevalence and economic costs in the community globally, the profound clinical effects on an individual's cognitive and general functioning and the increased risk of adverse health complications [2]. Moreover, mounting evidence suggests that OSA can increase the risk of cardiovascular diseases (hypertension, coronary heart failure, stroke etc.), metabolic syndrome, Neurological problems and increased in societal effects such as traffic accidents [3, 5–7].

2. Prevalence of OSA

OSA is a common chronic disorder with an estimated prevalence of 2–4% in general and the disorder was believed to be rising continuously with an approximate rate of 14% in men and 5% in women aged 30–70 years respectively [8–10]. It is higher in patients with obesity; diabetes mellitus type II and other cardiovascular disorders which includes ischemic heart disease, heart failure, cardiac arrhythmias, stroke, atherosclerosis and myocardial infarction [8, 10]. Research on current prevalence (Seventh Joint National Committee) shows that OSA was identified as a secondary cause of Hypertension (HTN) and ranges from 37 to 56%, the prevalence rate of OSA in resistant hypertensive patients were estimated to be 70–83% [11]. Among the pediatric population, the rate affects between 1.2 and 5.7% and it is estimated that 36% of obese children are at high risk of OSA [12]. Since it is reported that more than 85% of patients with OSA symptoms have never been diagnosed clinically [13].

3. Pathophysiology of OSA

The pathogenesis of OSA can be multifactorial, complex and incompletely understood [13, 14]. The changes in upper airway anatomy tissue characteristics and neuromuscular function, sleep-dependent changes can assume to play the major role between the individuals (**Figure 1**). Certain factors that may contribute to OSA include obesity, thickened lateral pharyngeal walls, nasal congestion, enlarged uvula, facial malformations, and tonsillar hypertrophy. As the patient falls asleep, the muscle tone of the nasopharynx is reduced during sleep and airways become contracted. These episodes are typically accompanied by repeated oxyhemoglobin desaturation, oxygen levels in the body start to drop and carbon dioxide levels rise by short micro-arousals by the patient when the airway patency is restored. This causes activation in sympathetic nervous system and contraction of nasopharyngeal tissue, which results in obstruction of the airway. These cyclic episodes continue throughout the night with reduced deep Non-Rapid eye movement sleep (NREM) and Rapid eye movement sleep (REM) [13]. Several studies have confirmed that the airway dilating muscles in OSA patients can no longer resist the negative pressure in airways during inspiration. In severe cases, the respiratory events can occur 50–100 times per hour; each event lasts for about 20–40 s [9].The severity of OSA is measured by the apnea-hypopnea index (AHI). The frequency of apneas and hypopneas per hour of sleep. Apnea is defined by complete obstruction of the upper airways lasting for at least 10 s (i.e. airflow restriction by more than 90% (according to AASM criteria). Hypopnea is defined as airflow restriction more than 30% (according to AASM criteria)

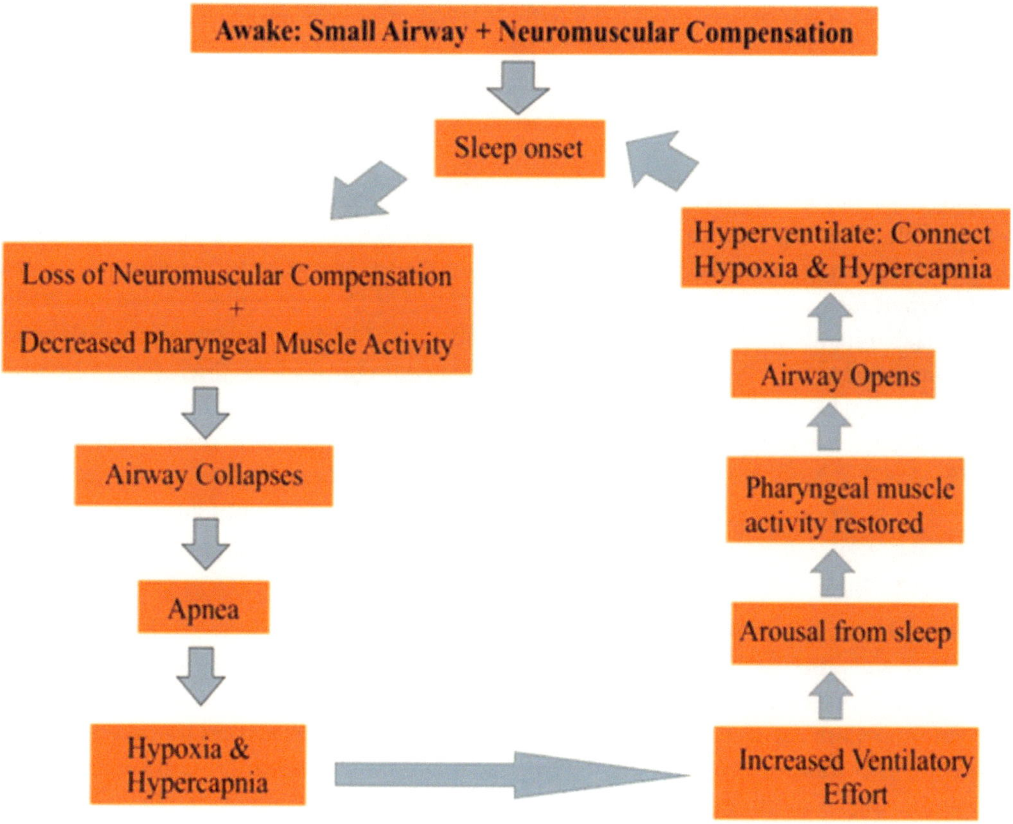

Figure 1. Pathophysiology of OSA.

OSA severity	RDI measurement (events/hr)
Mild OSA	≥ 5
Moderate OSA	≥ 15
Severe OSA	≥ 30

Table 1. OSA severity is defined by the AASM.

lasting for more than 10s. The oxygen desaturation index (ODI) is defined as the number of desaturations per 1 h of monitored sleep when oxygen saturation is reduced as compared to the baseline standard level. The respiratory effort related arousal (RERA) can also be used. RERA is defined as an episode characterized by an increased respiratory effort caused by upper airway airflow reduction resolved with arousal and accompanied in most cases with hypoxemia. The respiratory disturbance index (RDI) is the sum of RERA and AHI [9, 15].

According to the third edition of the International Classification of Sleep Disorders (ICSD-3), obstructive sleep apnea (OSA) is defined as polysomnography derived obstructive respiratory disturbance index (RDI) ≥5 events/h associated with typical OSA symptoms, or an obstructive RDI ≥15/h in the absence of clinical OSA symptoms [9]. According to American Academy of sleep medicine (AASM), OSA is commonly divided into three levels of severity as detailed in **Table 1** below.

4. Diagnosis of OSA

The diagnosis of Obstructive sleep apnea starts with thorough history and physical examination to elucidate the signs and symptoms of the syndrome. Common symptoms patients complain of snoring, disturbed sleep, daytime somnolence, decreased libido as well as a history of hypertension, cardiovascular disease, and diabetes. Depending on the nonspecific and other variable features of OSA, its diagnosis based on a clinician's subjective analysis alone may be inaccurate [13]. A number of out-patient screening questionnaires such as Epworth sleepiness scale (ESS), Berlin Questionnaire STOP-BANG questionnaire, Sleep Apnea of Sleep Disorder Questionnaire SA-SDQ, OSA50 questionnaire etc. to help and identify patients with OSA [9, 16, 17]. Advances in sleep medicine and the availability of improved diagnostic tools have led to a better recognition and treatment of the disease. The outpatient examination should be repeated and the patients should be then referred, depending on the result of the follow-up examination, to a sleep laboratory [8].

An overnight polysomnography is considered to be the gold standard for the diagnosis of obstructive sleep apnea (**Figures 1** and **2**). A screening tool is necessary to stratify patients based on their clinical symptoms, their physical examinations, and their risk factors, in order to ascertain patients at high risk and in urgent need of PSG and/or further treatment [18]. The diagnostic PSG was performed using the computerized polysomnographic system including the monitoring of electroencephalogram (EEG), submental and anterior tibial electromyogram (EMG), oxygen saturation (SaO_2), electrocardiogram (ECG), inductance plethysmography

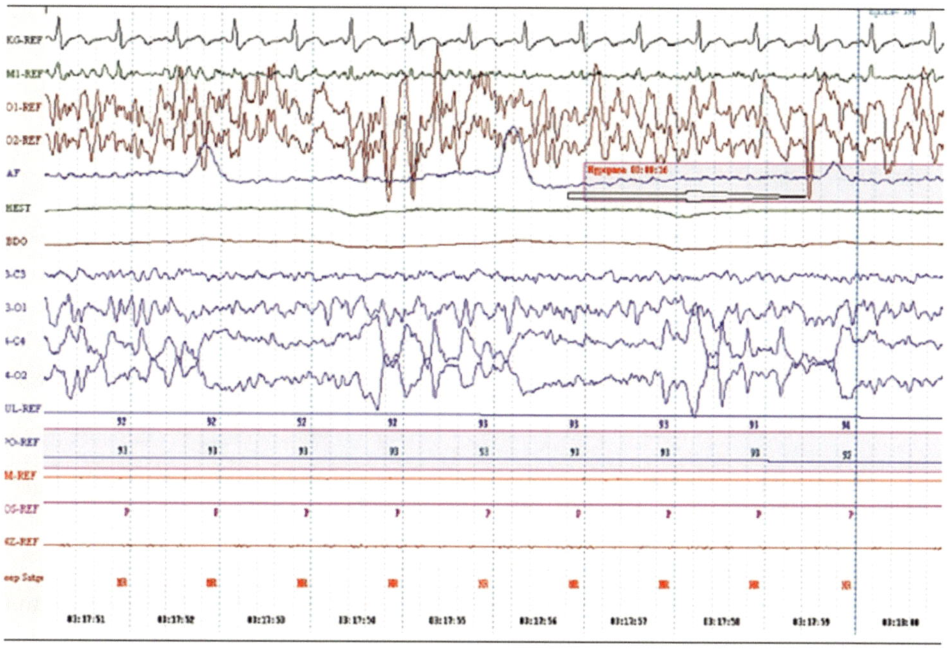

Figure 2. Polysomnography representation of airflow obstruction.

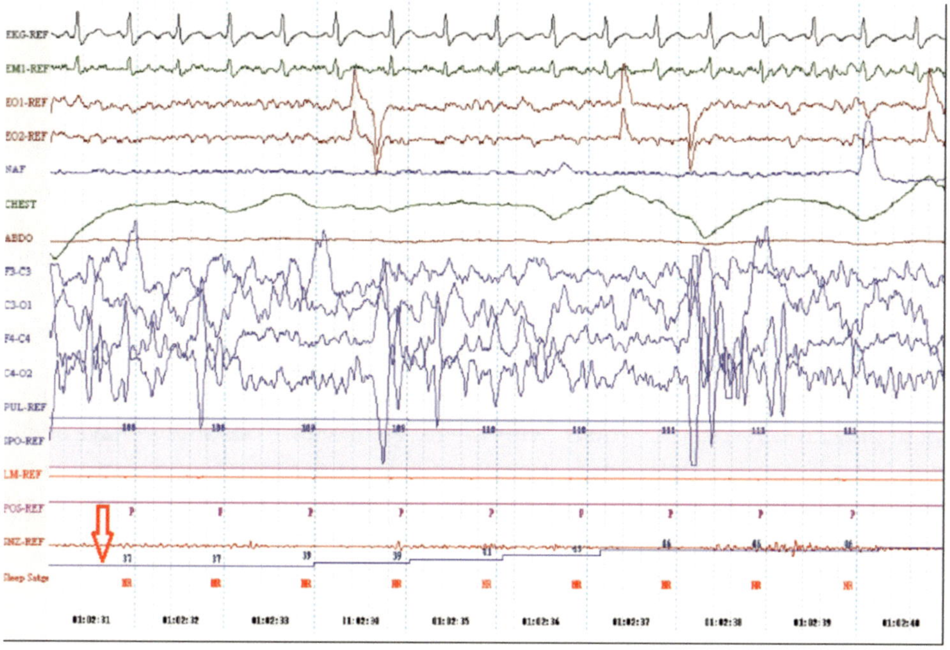

Figure 3. Polysomnography representation of airflow obstruction with desaturation.

of chest walls and abdomen, nasal pressure sensor, and oronasal thermistor. The polysomnographic recording was scored manually by the sleep specialist. The sleep stage scoring and event scoring were done in accordance with the American Academy of Sleep Medicine (AASM) Manual for the Scoring of Sleep and Associated Events [19] (**Figure 3**).

Total obstructive Apnea/hypopnea index (AHI) was calculated as the number of obstructive apneas and hypopneas per hour of total sleep time (TST). The threshold for diagnosis of OSA was set at an AHI ≥5 and the severity of OSA was arbitrarily defined by cut-off levels of AHI [20]. Additional diagnostic models for OSA include portable sleep monitors, radiographic studies for anatomic analysis. It is necessary to remember that OSA can occur and progress over short periods of time, and its association with significant morbidity, coupled with the relatively low risk and high reward of therapy, that requires a thorough workup and treatment plan [13].

5. Complications of OSA

Several risk factors have been identified in the development of OSA namely male gender(up to age 65), increasing age, menopause, overweight, truncal obesity reflected by several markers including BMI, neck circumference, and waist-to-hip ratio, craniofacial abnormalities, upper airway anatomy, smoking, alcohol, and genetic predisposition [21]. Obesity is considered as the most important clinical risk factor for the development of OSA. Several studies have shown that more than half of the prevalence of OSA is attributable to excess body weight as opposed to substantial improvement with weight reduction [19]. Fat Deposition around the pharyngeal airway and abdomen may likely to reduce residual capacity function, which would be predicted to reduce lung volume tethering effects on the upper airway [22]. This latter mechanism emphasizes the great importance of central obesity as compared with peripheral obesity since it is the abdomen much more than the thighs that affect upper-airway size. Therefore, obesity has been associated with functional impairment in upper airway muscles [23]. **Figure 4** represents the complications of OSA.

The prevalence of OSA increases with age and the gender differences diminish significantly after menopause [21]. Although several potential mechanisms have been proposed, the explanation for this aging increase in the prevalence of OSA remains unknown. The exact mechanism of OSA was not fully known but, it begins as just loud snoring, then gradually over a period of time cessations of breathing and symptoms of excessive sleepiness develop, and thereafter may remain stable or worsen with weight gain. Numerous studies have attempted to know the cause of the age-related impact on OSA, no definitive conclusions have been reached [22]. Anatomical and pathophysiological susceptibility to OSA appears to increase with age in older people, who had a poorer responsiveness of pharyngeal dilator muscles, the genioglossus negative pressure stimuli appear to deteriorate with aging [23].

Craniofacial anatomy is probably one of the important factors in non-obese cases with OSA. Several soft and hard tissue factors may alter the mechanical properties of the upper airway muscles and increase its propensity to collapse during sleep. Features such as retrognathia, tonsillar hypertrophy, soft palate, inferiorly positioned hyoid bone, maxillary and

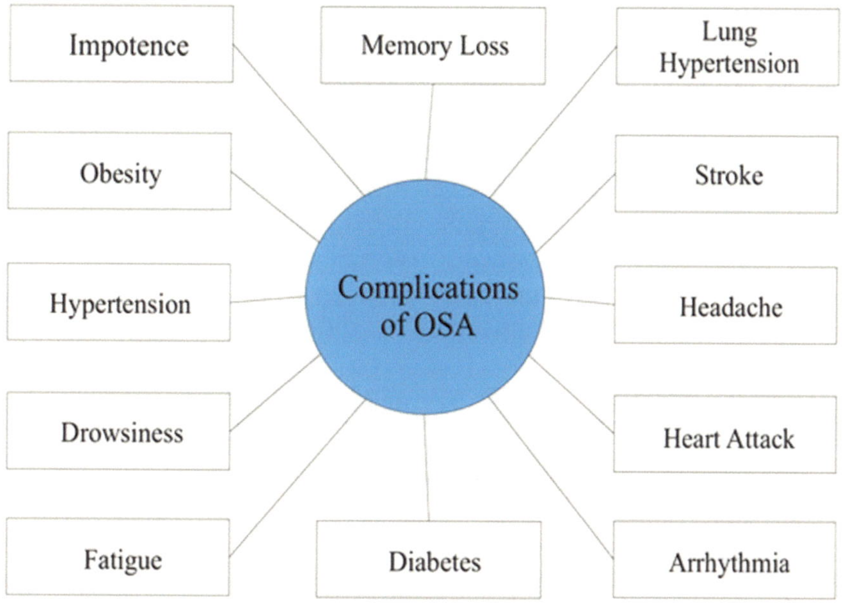

Figure 4. Complications of OSA.

mandibular retroposition, can narrow upper airway dimensions and promote the occurrence of apneas and hypopneas during sleep. Differences in craniofacial structures may alter the risk for obstructive sleep apnea across different racial groups. Therefore, different racial groups are prone to develop obstructive sleep apnea at varying degrees of obesity, clinicians should consider the possibility of this disorder particularly in the presence of clinically detectable craniofacial abnormalities [4]. According to clinic-based studies, the significant gender gap in the prevalence of OSA was reported. Recent population-based studies have confirmed that the prevalence of OSA is higher in men than women. This difference between clinic and epidemiological prevalence suggests several explanations for the gender gap. Firstly, women may not present with a similar symptomatic profile as men (loud snoring, nocturnal snorting or gasping, and witnessed apneas). Women were more likely to present with atypical complaints namely insomnia, depression, fatigue, and lack of energy, less likely to have apnea. The other reasons for this gender disparity are differences in body fat distribution (or other gender-related upper airway anatomy differences), control of ventilation, physiology of the pharyngeal airway dilator muscles activation, and hormonal differences. Therefore, the evidence suggests that women are underdiagnosed and untreated for OSA compared to men [21].

Social factors such as smoking and alcohol consumption are considered as possible risk factors for progression of obstructive symptoms [13]. Epidemiological studies show that current smoking is associated with high prevalence of snoring and obstructive sleep apnea. Smoking can alter the upper airway properties and increase its collapsibility during sleep [4]. Ingestion of alcohol especially at dinner or during the evening relaxes dilator muscles, increases upper airway resistance, and decreases respiratory reflexes, and so it leads to snoring and apnea episodes in susceptible individuals [24].

Familial aggregation of obstructive sleep apnea was first recognized in the 1970s by Strohl and co-workers in a family with several affected individuals. The relative risk of obstructive sleep apnea can be two-four fold higher in first-degree relatives [23]. Genetic factors of obesity, soft tissue characteristics, and craniofacial abnormalities together given the wealth of evidence implicating these factors in the pathogenesis of the disorder. However, the genetic basis of obstructive sleep apnea needs a better attention, the available study reports suggest that inquires about family history can help the clinician to diagnose the disorder early for further treatment [4].Medications such as muscle relaxants, sedative hypnotics (benzodiazepines and barbiturates), narcotics, opioid analgesics and other central nervous system depressants, preferentially inhibit upper airway muscle activity while also depressing the respiratory centers of the brain [24].

There are several other risk factors associated with OSA namely nasal congestion, pregnancy, menopause, hypothyroidism, diabetes and pregnancy. Available data suggest that OSA is three times higher in patients with insulin resistance than it is in the general population. Hypothyroidism leads to deposition of mucoproteins in the upper airway that causes enlargement of the soft palate, pharyngeal and laryngeal mucous membranes, thereby increasing the propensity for upper airway collapse during sleep. Thus, patients with hypothyroidism may have increased susceptibility to obstructive sleep apnea. Pregnant women also experience higher rates of snoring particularly in the third trimester due to some of the physiologic changes that accompany pregnancy (e.g., higher progesterone levels, decrease in sleep time in the supine position). Thus, early case identification may have implications for maternal and fetal outcomes. Knowledge of risk factors for obstructive sleep apnea is therefore crucial for proper diagnosis and treatment at those with the highest risk [4, 21].

6. Pharmacotherapy of OSA

OSA is a common condition in which nasal and oral airway ceases in spite of continued diaphragmatic efforts and is associated with poor quality of life, increased healthcare-related costs. Numerous efficacious treatments are available, but the patient should not shy away from therapeutic options, and medical practitioners should not hesitate to implement treatment regimens in addressing the problem of OSA. Treatment of OSA depends on the severity, duration, and cause of the patient's symptoms as well as the patient's lifestyle, comorbidities, and overall health [13]. The detailed treatment procedures are discussed below (**Figure 5**):

6.1. Positive airway pressure treatment (PAP)

First-line therapy for most patients with OSA continues the use of PAP especially in patients with greater apnea-hypopnea index score (AHI). PAP devices work as pneumatic support that allows maintaining adequate airway patency above a critical value (pressure value below which the airway collapses). The device is applied to the patient, through a nasal or oronasal mask during sleep in overnight at a required positive pressure. The pressure

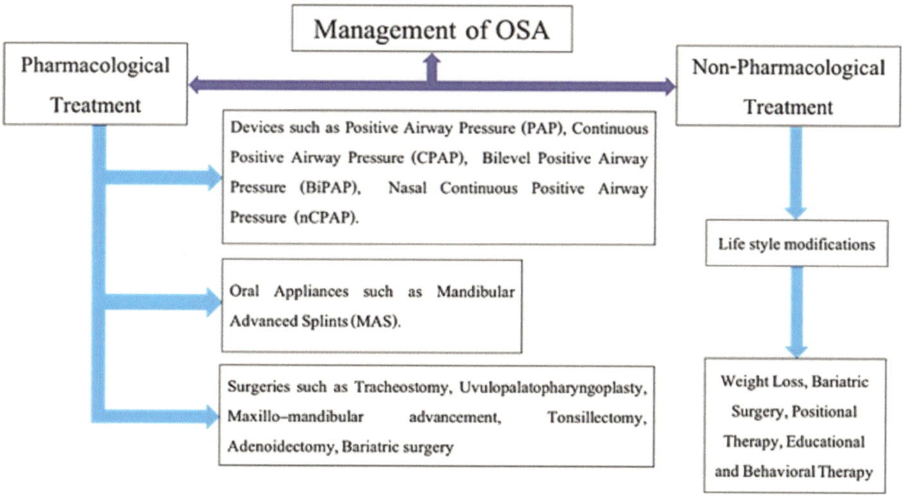

Figure 5. Pharmacotherapy of OSA.

can be varying with the severity of OSA and high pressures are required to avoid apneas during rapid eye movement sleep (REM) in the supine position or in severe obesity cases. However, patient compliance for PAP devices levels average 40–50% due to mask leaks, nasal congestion and sleep disruption. In moderate to severe OSA cases PAP therapy is remains as life-long treatment, many advanced PAP ventilators such as continuous positive airway pressure (CPAP), auto-titrating positive airway pressure (APAP), and bi-level positive airway pressure (BPAP) therapies have been commercialized in order to maintain efficacy and maximal comfort for patients [8, 25].

6.2. Continuous positive airway pressure (CPAP)

CPAP therapy was initially applied as treatment of OSA by Sullivan and colleagues in 1981 [26]. Since its initial description, the device is considered as the gold standard treatment for OSA. The clinical application of this CPAP has deeply modified the course of the disease over the last three decades, offering to thousands of patients the first non-invasive method to control their disorder. Worldwide, CPAP is constantly recommended as the first-choice treatment for patients with moderate to severe OSA. Continuous PAP (CPAP), generally administered through the nose (nCPAP), delivers a single pressure to the posterior pharynx throughout the night and acts as a pneumatic splint that maintains the patency of the upper airway in a dose-dependent fashion. The best pressure for CPAP treatment is typically determined during an in-laboratory attended sleep study. CPAP therapy is indicated in all patients with an AHI greater than 15, independently from the presence of comorbidities, type of work and severity of symptoms; if the AHI is above 5 and below 15, CPAP is indicated in the presence of symptoms (i.e. sleepiness, impaired cognition, mood disorders) or in the presence of hypertension, coronary artery disease or previous cerebrovascular accidents [8, 25, 27].

6.3. Oral appliances

Over the last 10 years, oral appliances have gained increasing recognition as a useful alternative to CPAP for the treatment of patients with mild to moderate OSA and for those who do not tolerate or adhere to CPAP. The most frequently used oral appliances are mandibular advanced splints (MAS). These splints attach to both the upper and lower dental arches in order to advance and retain the mandible in a forward position, further the size of upper airway will be widened particularly in its lateral dimension, and the function of upper airway dilator muscles, particularly the genioglossus, will improve through the protrusion of the jaw during sleep [30]. As the pharyngeal collapsibility is reduced, the risk of apnoeic events will be lowered. Side effects that are more persistent include arthralgia, teeth pain and occlusal changes [8]. Several randomized trials have evaluated the efficacy of MAS versus CPAP in mild to moderate obstructive sleep apnea, treatment with MAS significantly reduces the number of apneas/hypopneas (normalizing nocturnal SaO2), reduces daytime somnolence, and improves quality of life [28]. It has been demonstrated that the treatment success is achieved in patients with the following characteristics: young people, women, patients with small necks, and milder OSA [29]. Another group of oral appliances includes the orthodontic micro-implants that are connected to the extra-orally anchored mask. Overnight application of these devices significantly reduces the AHI and few studies have shown similar efficacy compared with MAS. This type of implants could be used in patients with few teeth, exaggerated gag reflex, or intolerance for classic MADs [27]. Although its efficacy is still undetermined to recommend the use of these oral appliances in clinical practice [30].

The role of surgery in the management of OSA has been widely explored in an attempt to find a treatment option that could be definitive [6]. A wide variety of procedures are available, many of which are directed at the site of obstruction [2]. Initially, Kuhlo and colleagues in 1969 followed by Lugaresi and colleagues in 1970 were the first to treat OSA effectively (or Pickwickian syndrome) by means of a tracheostomy. By bypassing the upper airway, tracheostomy is purported to be curative for OSA. The surgical procedure is effective at preventing OSA-related arrhythmias, reducing pulmonary artery pressures, and improving hypertension and diabetes in patients with OSA. Unfortunately, tracheostomy has several problems including patient dissatisfaction (e.g., psychosocial aspects), perioperative complications (e.g., wound infection, tissue necrosis, bleeding), recurrent bronchitis, granulation tissue, trachea-innominate fistula formation, and stoma stenosis [31].

6.4. Surgical treatment

The aim of the surgery is to remove the cause of upper airway obstruction and to widen the airway, after a precise detection of the site where the obstruction occurs [8]. The most common sites of obstruction are the oropharyngeal tract (collapse of the retropalatal and retrolingual regions due to macroglossia, low-lying soft palate or enlarged tonsils) and the nose (congestion, polyposis, chronic rhinitis) [32]. Tonsillectomy and adenoidectomy are the most commonly used surgical procedures to treat OSA in children and are highly effective [8]. Uvulopalatopharyngoplasty (UPPP), either conventional or laser assisted (LAPP), is a widely used surgical procedure for the treatment of OSA. This technique consists of the resection of the uvula, part of the soft palate and tissue excess in the oropharynx, and is usually performed with simultaneous tonsillectomy [31]. The success rate for UPPP alone is 30, 60% along with a tonsillectomy. The common side effects of UPPP surgery include velopharyngeal insufficiency (up to one-third of patients), dry throat and swallowing difficulty [33]. Tracheotomy is the most established surgical treatment for OSA and must be carried out in selected patients with severe OSA for whom all other treatment approaches have failed [34]. Maxillomandibular advancement (MMA) is indeed a highly effective treatment for tracheotomy. In fact, the efficacy of most treatments decreases with age and weight gain. This indicates a major factor determining the recurrence of OSA after surgery [8].

6.5. Weight control and bariatric surgery

Excess body weight and obesity are considered as largest predisposing factors for obstructive sleep apnea (OSA) over 70% of OSA patients have obesity. Population-based studies have documented a strong correlation between body mass index (BMI) and apnea-hypopnea index (AHI). Observational studies on the effects of dietary or surgical weight loss which show that reducing obstructive sleep apnea severity is possible with a decrease in body weight where a significant reduction in AHI score can be seen [4]. In patients with morbid obesity (BMI > 40) bariatric surgery, including gastric bypass and bandage, is presented as the optimal alternative for achieving considerable weight reduction when conservative treatments like CPAP, oral devices, and upper airway surgeries are failed [35]. Evidence has demonstrated, that bariatric surgery is co-adjuvant in the treatment of OSA, effectively reducing severity in up to 75% of cases. But, the remission rate for OSA 2 years after bariatric surgery in relation to the quantity of weight loss is up to 40% [27].

6.6. Educational and behavioral therapies

Educational and behavioral therapies are the first step in approaching patients with OSA, independently from the treatment chosen. Patients should be instructed to avoid risk factors such as tobacco, alcohol consumption (particularly in the evening), using sedatives and hypnotics. The physician main priority is to explain the patients the role that obesity plays in their disorder, and advice to maintain an optimal weight [8]. Another goal of the educational therapy is to help each patient to recognize the need for regular use of nocturnal CPAP. Recent reports suggest that a supportive intervention can significantly increase compliance in patients with moderate to severe OSA [36].

6.7. Positional therapy

Body position during sleep greatly affects the number and severity of obstructive events due to anatomical and physiological mechanisms. The supine position, mainly due to effects of the gravity on the tongue and soft palate position, is generally associated with an increased number of apneas/hypopneas [37]. Postural OSA can take place mainly in patients sleeping in the supine position. If postural OSA is diagnosed with standard criteria, patients can benefit from a positional therapy (PT). The therapy includes "Tennis ball technique" consisting of a tennis ball strapped to the back to discourage supine position, supine alarm devices and a number of positional pillows. The success rate can be considered by proper selection of patients and post-treatment AHI has to below 10. However, trials on the long-term effects of PT on important outcomes, such as metabolic and neurocognitive changes, are still need to be studied [38].

A number of novel therapeutic options for management of obstructive sleep apnea are now under evaluation. The stimulation of upper airway muscles has been considered as a potential approach to prevent obstructive apneas over the years [39]. The Inspire Upper Airway Stimulation is the first system recently approved in patients with moderate to severe OSA, who are intolerant to use CPAP. Trials conducted on patients with moderate to severe OSA intolerant to CPAP showed 68% reduction in the median AHI score with a subjective improvement in daytime sleepiness and quality of life over 12 months of period [40]. Other emerging treatment options are intended for patients with mild disease or as a remedy for simple snoring. Among these nasal expiratory PAP (nEPAP) has recently gained attention [41]. The nEPAP is a disposable adhesive device placed over each nostril in order to increase the airflow resistance during the exhalation with a consequent improvement in the upper airway patency. A study in patients with mild to moderate OSA, nEPAP significantly reduce apneas, snoring, AHI score and improves subjective daytime sleepiness [42]. Therefore, further research is necessary to assess the potential benefits of this evolving technology.

7. Conclusion

Over recent decades, diverse studies have carried out to improve our understanding of the physiological mechanisms and outcomes of OSA, providing relevant insights into its potential contribution to the development of various treatment alternatives. Although an effective treatment is still unavailable, the combination of several therapeutic strategies to prevent of risk factors, improving sleep disturbance and quality of life should be the focus in patients with OSA. A multidisciplinary approach is needed for a treatment protocol that is able to directly address the etiological processes of the disease in order to reduce its prevalence.

Acknowledgements

We would like to thank Dr. T. Ramphanindra, Post Graduate in Respiratory Medicine.

Conflict of interest

We wish to confirm that there are no known conflicts of interest associated with this publication.

Author details

Jyothi I[1]*, Renuka Prasad K[2], Rajalakshmi R[3], Satish Kumar RC[1], Ramphanindra Talatam[4], Vijayakumar TM[2] and Kaliappan Ilango[1]

*Address all correspondence to: jyothiinampudi@gmail.com

1 Clinical Trial and Research Unit, Interdisciplinary Institute of Indian System of Medicine (IIISM), SRM Institute of Science and Technology, Kattankulathur, Kanchipuram (DT), Tamil Nadu, India

2 Department of Pharmacy Practice, SRM College of Pharmacy, SRM Institute of Science and Technology, Kattankulathur, Kanchipuram (DT), Tamil Nadu, India

3 Department of Respiratory Medicine, SRM Medical College Hospital and Research Centre, SRM Institute of Science and Technology, Kattankulathur, Kanchipuram (DT), Tamil Nadu, India

4 Department of Pulmonary Medicine, SRM Medical College Hospital and Research Centre, SRM Institute of Science and Technology, Kattankulathur, Kanchipuram (DT), Tamil Nadu, India

References

[1] Paskhover B. An introduction to obstructive sleep apnea. Otolaryngologic Clinics of North America. 2016;**49**:1303-1306. DOI: 10.1016/j.otc.2016.07.007

[2] Qureshi A, Ballard RD. Obstructive sleep apnea. The Journal of Allergy and Clinical Immunology. 2003;**112**:643-651. DOI: 10.1016/j.jaci.2003.08.031

[3] Xia Y, Fu Y, Xu H, Guan J, Yi H, Yin S. Changes in cerebral metabolites in obstructive sleep apnea: A systemic review and meta-analysis. Scientific Reports. 2016;**6**:28712. DOI: 10.1038/srep28712

[4] Punjabi NM. The epidemiology of adult obstructive sleep apnea. Proceedings of the American Thoracic Society. 2008;**5**:136-143. DOI: 10.1513/pats.200709-155MG

[5] Scarlata S, Pennazza G, Santonico M, Santangelo S, Rossi Bartoli I, Rivera C, Vernile C, Vincentis AD, Incalzi RA. Screening of obstructive sleep apnea syndrome by electronic-nose analysis of volatile organic compounds. Scientific Reports. 2017;**7**:11938. DOI: 10.1038/s41598-017-12108-w

[6] Cao C, Wu B, Wu Y, Yu Y, Ma H, Sun S, Zhang Q, Ding Q, Chen L, Deng Z. Functional polymorphisms in the promoter region of MMP-2 and MMP-9 and susceptibility to obstructive sleep apnea. Scientific Reports. 2015;**5**:8966. DOI: 10.1038/srep08966

[7] Fornadi K, Ronai KZ, Turanyi CZ, Malavade TS, Shapiro CM, Novak M, Mucsi I, Molnar MZ. Sleep apnea is not associated with worse outcomes in kidney transplant recipients. Scientific Reports. 2014;**4**:6987. DOI: 10.1038/srep06987

[8] Spicuzza L, Caruso D, Di Maria G. Obstructive sleep apnoea syndrome and its management. Therapeutic Advances in Chronic Disease. 2015;**6**(5):273-285. DOI:10.1177/2040622315590318

[9] Kamasova M, Vaclavik J, Taborsky M. Obstructive sleep apnea in outpatient care – What to do with? Cor et Vasa. 2017:e 1-e 7. DOI: 10.1016/j.crvasa.2017.09.004

[10] Drager LF, Togeiro SM, Polotsky VY, Lorenzi-Filho G. Obstructive sleep apnea: A cardiometabolic risk in obesity and the metabolic syndrome. Journal of the American College of Cardiology. 2013;**62**:569-576. DOI: 10.1016/j.jacc.2013.05.045

[11] Pedrosa RP, Drager LF, Gonzaga CC, Sousa MG, de Paula LKG, Amaro ACS, Amodeo C, Bortolotto LA, Krieger EM, Douglas Bradley T, Lorenzi-Filho G. Obstructive sleep apnea the most common secondary cause of hypertension associated with resistant hypertension. Hypertension. 2011;**58**:811-817. DOI: 10.1161/HYPERTENSIONAHA.111.179788

[12] Brockbank JC. Update on pathophysiology and treatment of childhood obstructive sleep apnea syndrome. Pediatric Respiratory Reviews. 2017;**24**:21-23. DOI: 10.1016/j.prrv.2017.06.003

[13] Motamedi KK, McClary AC, Amedee RG. Obstructive sleep apnea: A growing problem. The Ochsner Journal. 2009;**9**:149-153

[14] Deegan PC, McNicholas WT. Pathophysiology of obstructive sleep apnoea. European Respiratory Journal. 1995;**8**:1161-1178

[15] Ramar K, Dort LC, Katz SG, Lettieri CJ, Harrod CG, Thomas SM, Chervin RD. Clinical practice guideline for the treatment of obstructive sleep apnea and snoring with oral appliance therapy: An update for 2015. Journal of Clinical Sleep Medicine: Official Publication of the American Academy of Sleep Medicine. 2015;**11**:773-827. DOI: 10.5664/jcsm.4858

[16] Hassan I. El-Sayed comparison of four sleep questionnaires for screening obstructive sleep apnea. Egyptian Journal of Chest Diseases and Tuberculosis. 2012;**61**:433-441. DOI: 10.1016/j.ejcdt.2012.07.003

[17] Prasad KT, Sehgal IS, Agarwal R, Nath Aggarwal A, Behera D, Dhooria S. Assessing the likelihood of obstructive sleep apnea: A comparison of nine screening questionnaires. Sleep & Breathing. 2017;**21**:909-917. DOI: 10.1007/s11325-017-1495-4

[18] Abrishami A, Khajehdehi A, Chung F. A systematic review of screening questionnaires for obstructive sleep apnea. Canadian Journal of Anaesthesia. 2010;**57**:423-438. DOI: 10.1007/s12630-010-9280-x

[19] Preethi P, Arvin Kumar C, Reddy G, Chandrasekhar C, Rajagopalan B. Comparison of three sleep questionnaires in screening obstructive sleep apnoea. Journal of Evolution of Medical and dental sciences. 2017;**88**:6132-6136. DOI: 10.14260/jemds/2017/1332

[20] Health Quality Ontario. Polysomnography in patients with obstructive sleep apnea: An evidence-based analysis. Ontario Health Technology Assessment Series. 2006;**6**:1-38

[21] Lee W, Nagubadi S, Kryger MH, Mokhlesi B. Epidemiology of obstructive sleep apnea: A population-based perspective. Expert Review of Respiratory Medicine. 2008;**2**(3):349-364. DOI: 10.1586/17476348.2.3.349

[22] Eckert DJ, Malhotra A. Pathophysiology of adult obstructive sleep apnea.Proceedings of the American Thoracic Society. 2008;**5**:144-153. DOI:10.1513/pats.200707-114MG

[23] Pillar G, Lavie P. Obstructive Sleep Apnea: Diagnosis, Risk Factors, and Pathophysiology. In: Montagna P, Chokroverty S, editors. Handbook of Clinical Neurology

[24] Paiva T, Attarian H. Obstructive sleep apnea, and other sleep-related syndromes. In: Biller J, Ferro MJ, editors. Handbook of Clinical Neurology

[25] Freedman N. Treatment of obstructive sleep apnea: Choosing the best positive airway pressure device. Sleep Medicine Clinics. 2017;**12**:529-542. DOI: 10.1016/j.jsmc.2017.07.003

[26] Sullivan C, Berthon-Jones M, Issa F. Nocturnal nasal-airway pressure for sleep apnea. The New England Journal of Medicine. 1983;**309**:112. DOI: 10.1056/NEJM198307143090215

[27] Cortes-Reyes E, Parrado-Bermudez K, Escobar-Cordoba F. New perspectives in the treatment of obstructive sleep apnea-hypopnea syndrome. Colombian Journal of Anesthesiology. 2017;**45**:62-71. DOI: https://doi.org/10.1016/j.rcae.2016.07.002

[28] Vanderveken OM, Devolder A, Marklund M, Boudewyns AN, Braem MJ, Okkerse W, Verbraecken JA, Franklin KA, De Backer WA, Van de Heyning PH. Comparison of a custom-made and a thermoplastic oral appliance for the treatment of mild sleep apnea. American Journal of Respiratory and Critical Care Medicine. 2008;**178**:197-202. DOI: 10.1164/rccm.200701-114OC

[29] Mehta A, Qian J, Petocz P, Darendeliler MA, Cistulli PA. A randomized, controlled study of a mandibular advancement splint for obstructive sleep apnea. American Journal of Respiratory and Critical Care Medicine. 2001;**163**:1457-1461. DOI: 10.1164/ajrccm.163.6.2004213

[30] Randerath WJ, Verbraecken J, Andreas S, Bettega G, Boudewyns A, Hamans E, Jalbert F, Paoli JR, Sanner B, Smith I, Stuck BA, Lacassagne L, Marklund M, Maurer JT, Pepin JL, Valipour A, Verse T, Fietze I. European Respiratory Society task force on non-CPAP therapies in sleep apnoea. Non-CPAP therapies in obstructive sleep apnoea. The European Respiratory Journal. 2011;**37**:1000-1028. DOI: 10.1183/09031936.00099710

[31] Holty J-EC, Guilleminault C. Surgical options for the treatment of obstructive sleep apnea. The Medical clinics of North America. 2010;**94**:479-515

[32] Dempsey JA, Veasey SC, Morgan BJ, O'Donnell CP. Pathophysiology of sleep apnea. Physiological Reviews. 2010;**90**:47-112. DOI: 10.1152/physrev.00043.2008

[33] Verse T, Hormann K. The surgical treatment of sleep-related upper airway obstruction. Deutsches Arzteblatt International. 2011;**108**:216-221. DOI: 10.3238/arztebl.2010.0216

[34] Epstein LJ, Kristo D, Strollo PJ, Friedman N, Malhotra A, Patil SP, Ramar K, Rogers R, Schwab RJ, Weaver EM, Weinstein MD. Adult obstructive sleep apnea task force of the

American Academy of sleep medicine. Clinical guideline for the evaluation, management and long-term care of obstructive sleep apnea in adults. Journal of Clinical Sleep Medicine: JCSM: Official Publication of the American Academy of Sleep Medicine. 2009;**5**:263-276

[35] Sarkhosh K, Switzer NJ, El-Hadi M, Birch DW, Shi X, Karmali S. The impact of bariatric surgery on obstructive sleep apnea: A systematic review. Obesity Surgery. 2013;**23**:414-423. DOI: 10.1007/s11695-012-0862-2

[36] Wozniak DR, TJJ L, Smith I. Educational, supportive and behavioral interventions to improve usage of continuous positive airway pressure machines in adults with obstructive sleep apnoea. The Cochrane Database of Systematic Reviews. 2014:CD007736. DOI: 10.1002/14651858.CD007736.pub2

[37] Bidarian-Moniri A, Nilsson M, Rasmusson L, Attia J, Ejnell H. The effect of the prone sleeping position on obstructive sleep apnoea. Acta Oto-Laryngologica. 2015;**135**:79-84. DOI: 10.3109/00016489.2014.962183

[38] Frank MH, Ravesloot MJL, van Maanen JP, Verhagen E, de Lange J, de Vries N. Positional OSA part 1: Towards a clinical classification system for position-dependent obstructive sleep apnoea. Sleep and Breathing. 2015;**19**:473-480. DOI: 10.1007/s11325-014-1022-9

[39] Dedhia RC, Strollo PJ, Soose RJ. Upper airway stimulation for obstructive sleep apnea: Past, present, and future. Sleep. 2015;**38**:899-906. DOI: 10.5665/sleep.4736

[40] Strollo PJJ, Soose RJ, Maurer JT, de Vries N, Cornelius J, Froymovich O, Hanson RD, Padhya TA, Steward DL, Gillespie MB, Woodson BT, Van de Heyning PH, Goetting MG, Vanderveken OM, Feldman N, Knaack L, Strohl KP, STAR Trial Group. Upper-airway stimulation for obstructive sleep apnea. The New England Journal of Medicine. 2014;**370**:139-149. DOI: 10.1056/NEJMoa1308659

[41] Freedman N. Improvements in current treatments and emerging therapies for adult obstructive sleep apnea. F1000 Prime Reports. 2014;**6**:36. DOI: 10.12703/P6-36

[42] Kryger MH, Berry RB, Massie CA. Long-term use of a nasal expiratory positive airway pressure (EPAP) device as a treatment for obstructive sleep apnea (OSA). Journal of Clinical Sleep Medicine: JCSM: Official Publication of the American Academy of Sleep Medicine. 2011;**7**:449-53B. DOI: 10.5664/JCSM.1304

Chapter 3

Noninvasive Ventilation in Neuromuscular Diseases

Lavinia Davidescu, Diana Manolescu,
Ruxandra Ulmeanu and Cristian Oancea

Additional information is available at the end of the chapter

http://dx.doi.org/10.5772/intechopen.77173

Abstract

Respiratory muscle weakness is the main contributor to respiratory imbalance in patients with neuromuscular diseases (NMD). In the advanced stages of the disease, patients develop a chronic respiratory failure due to muscle weakness, which is the principal cause of death among these patients. Respiratory muscle weakness ultimately causes alveolar hypoventilation, initially nocturnal, and later daytime respiratory failure. The signs and symptoms of early respiratory muscle weakness are discrete, namely: dyspnoea on effort, orthopnea, insomnia, frequent nocturnal awakenings, morning headache, loss of appetite, excessive daytime sleepiness, depression, anxiety, and marked fatigue. The management of respiratory failure in neuromuscular diseases requires the use of non-invasive ventilation (NIV) to assist the respiratory muscles in order to correct the alveolar hypoventilation and ameliorate gas exchange. NIV thus slows down the decline of forced vital capacity thereby improving the patient's quality of life, physical activity and hemodynamics, normalization of blood gases, slight improvement in other physiological measures, and maximal mouth pressures and increases survival. NIV support should be offered to all patients who present with early signs of ventilatory failure as it is probably the most effective among treatments in prolonging life in neuromuscular patients.

Keywords: non-invasive ventilation, respiratory failure, neuromuscular diseases

1. Introduction

Neuromuscular diseases (NMD) are a group of diseases that affect the nerves that control voluntary muscles, including respiratory muscles in more advanced stages, that varies according to underlying disease [1]. The weakness of the respiratory muscles causes alveolar hypoventilation, initially during sleep, and then leading to respiratory insufficiency in the daytime [1, 6]. Respiratory infections, in which neuromuscular patients are predisposed, usually aggravate the evolution of respiratory insufficiency.

Muscle weakness affects three categories of muscles involved in breathing:

- Inspiratory muscles, which contribute to the act of ventilation and voluntary inspiration.
- Expiratory muscles performing forced expiration and forced expiratory flow.
- Bulbar muscles, which have a glottic function, thus contributing to swallowing/speech, increased intra-thoracic pressure and cough [4, 9, 13].

Affection of inspiring muscles in NMD leads to dyspnoea, orthopnea, alveolar hypoventilation and hypercapnia. Alveolar hypoventilation occurs initially during rapid eyes movement sleep (REM) sleep, then in non-REM sleep, leading to morning hypercapnia and later in the evening hypercapnia as well as hypoxia [2, 3, 8, 13]. The weakness of the expiratory muscles leads to an inefficient clearance of the airway, ineffective cough, thus predisposing to respiratory infections. Affecting bulbar muscles causes swallowing and speech disturbances, aspiration secretions, reduced airway clearance, and recurrent respiratory infections [1, 6, 8, 13].

Existing studies have shown, mostly uncontrolled trials, that non-invasive ventilation (NIV) in neuromuscular diseases improved quality of life, physical activity and hemodynamic, normalization of blood gases and slight improvement in other physiological measures, such as the vital capacity and maximal mouth pressures [1, 3, 5, 6, 11, 12].

Monitoring of patients diagnosed with NMD is essential for the early detection of signs of respiratory failure and the establishment of NIV at an early stage of respiratory distress.

2. Signs and symptoms of respiratory failure in neuromuscular diseases

2.1. Symptoms

The symptoms of respiratory muscle weakness depend on the speed of its development. When the onset is subacute (for example, in Guillain-Barre syndrome), the predominant symptoms are dyspnoea and orthopnea, or sometimes respiratory arrest. These symptoms are often accompanied by those of bulbar weakness and inability to clear respiratory secretions. The symptoms of respiratory failure may easily be overlooked and should be specifically sought in any patient with rapidly progressive weakness, especially when the bulbar muscles and shoulder girdle are affected [4, 8, 9, 11].

When respiratory muscle weakness develops gradually, inadequate respiration usually occurs first during sleep. Symptoms of nocturnal hypoventilation include a broken sleep pattern, nightmares, nocturnal confusion, morning headache, daytime fatigue, mental clouding and somnolence [4, 8, 9, 11].

Symptoms	Signs
Dyspnea to minimal effort or speech	Tachypnea
Orthopnoea	The use of auxiliary respiratory muscles
Frequent nocturnal awakenings	Paradoxical abdominal movements
Excessive daytime sleepiness	Reducing the amplitude of the thoracic movements
Daytime fatigue	Ineffective cough
Morning headaches	Sweating
Difficulty to expectorate secretions	Tachycardia
Apathy, loss of appetite	Morning confusion, hallucination
Hypomnesic concentration deficiency and memory impairment	Weight loss
Difficulty sleeping	Dry mouth or hypersalivation

Table 1. Signs and symptoms of respiratory failure in neuromuscular diseases.

Rapidly progressive NMD	Variable progression	Slowly progressive or non-progressive
Amyotrophic lateral sclerosis (ALS)	Limb girdle muscular dystrophy	Spinal muscular atrophy
Duchene muscular dystrophy (DMD)	Miopathies Nemaline miopathy Metabolic miopathy	Poliomyelitis, post-polio syndrome
	Merosin negative congenital muscular distrophy	Facio-scapulohumeral muscular dystrophy
		Becker muscular dystrophy

Table 2. Classification of Neuromuscular disorders (NMD) according to evolution [1].

Exertional dyspnoea is encountered less frequently in neuromuscular patients than in those with other cardiorespiratory disorders, particularly when the patient has reduced mobility. Dyspnoea when lying flat or immersed in water specifically suggests weakness of diaphragm [4, 9].

2.2. Signs

A patient with severe respiratory muscle weakness or respiratory failure may appear overtly breathless and may be using accessory muscle of respiration. The patient may be unable to speak in complete sentences or take deep breaths to command. Inability to count from 1 to 20 in a single breath indicates significant reduction of vital capacity (VC) or forced vital capacity (FVC) [4, 9, 11]. Paradoxical abdominal motion (inwards movement of the abdominal wall with inspiration) suggests significant weakness of the diaphragm. The combination of hypoxemia and respiratory acidosis may produce mental clouding or somnolence. It is also important to assess the bulbar musculature, weakness of which can hinder clearing of respiratory secretions and so allow aspiration. Most of the patients with respiratory muscle weakness resulting from a neuromuscular condition have limb weakness. Acute respiratory failure in patients with neuromuscular disorders is often precipitated by respiratory infection [4, 8, 9, 11].

Particular attention should be paid to:

- Presence or absence of bulbar weakness.
- A tall, thin face (congenital myopathy, myotonic dystrophy)
- Ptosis of ophthalmoparesis (myasthenia)
- Fasciculation (motor neuron diseases)
- Paraspinal muscle wasting (acid maltase deficiency)
- Skin rash (dermatomyositis)

The main signs and symptoms of respiratory failure in the NMD can be found in **Tables 1** and **2**.

3. Course of neuromuscular disorders

Neuromuscular disorders can be divided into slowly progressive, rapidly progressive and NMD with variable progression; understanding the speed of progression of the disease is important in deciding the appropriateness of NIV [1, 2].

In the rapidly progressive NMD, the prototype of this category is Duchenne muscular dystrophy (DMD). Monitoring these patients begin in early ambulance stage, when the patient can walk independently, by using serial spirometry, sleep studies and blood gases, for capturing early FVC decline and respiratory disturbance in REM and non-REM sleep [11, 14].

In general, reducing FVC demonstrated by spirometry does not correlate very well with the occurrence of dyspnea as a symptom at these patients. Therefore, monitoring of clinical signs and symptoms of respiratory disturbance is not enough. Alveolar hypoventilation, secondary to respiratory muscular weakness, initially occurs in REM sleep, and it can be early diagnosed by using polysomnography. In a later stage, sleep disturbances occur both in REM and non-REM sleep, resulting in morning hypercapnia, and in the final stages, it also occurs during the daytime [11, 14].

The classical spirometry measuring FVC has some limitation in detecting moderate inspiratory muscle weakness; performing lung function test in supine position, could improve the value of FVC [16]. In DMD and other rapidly progressive NMD, initial evaluation using spirometry, polysomnography, blood gases and SaO2 is performed once a year, subsequently two times a year, and in advanced stages at 3 months [11, 14]. In slowly progression NMDs and those with variable progression, annual monitoring is sufficient.

4. Monitoring evolution of NMD

From a functional stand point, neuromuscular patients can be classified as following:

- Ambulant patients, who can walk without any help.
- Non-ambulant patients, who cannot stand seated without any help.
- Non-ambulant patients, who can stand seated without any help, but cannot walk without any help [14].

The monitoring of the patients is in relation with the specific neuromuscular disease and the rate of progression of the disease in each patient. It is recommended that the respiratory evaluation be done every 3–6 months, less frequently for ambulant patients, and more frequently for the nonambulant patients, and where the disease progresses at a faster pace.

Methods for respiratory monitoring in NMD:

- Spirometry
- Pulse oximetry
- Blood gases or capnography
- Polysomnography and/or cardiorespiratory polygraph
- Manometry for measurement of maximum inspiratory pressure (MIP) and maximum expiratory pressure (MEP)
- Cough peak flowmetry
- Sniff nasal inspiratory pressure (SNIP)

Spirometry and lung function testing are useful for detection of reducing FVC [11, 21] It can be applied while the patient is standing, however, classical spirometry measuring FVC has some limitations in detecting moderate inspiratory muscle weakness, spirometry in supine position is recommended. When measured FVC is in the supine position, vital capacity is lower, especially in patients with diaphragmatic weakness. Supine vital capacity may be useful in monitoring disease progression [11, 20]. A vital capacity of <1.11 liters predicted risk of chest infection with a sensitivity of 90.5% and a specificity of 70.8% [11].

Peak flowmetry during cough [cough peak expiratory flow (PEF)] allows efficient evaluation of coughing. A cough with PEF <270 ml/min suggests ineffective coughing [16].

Pulse oximetry can be used for highlighting hypoxemia during day, but also for guiding during the clearance of the airways. If the O_2 saturation is lower than 94%, clearance of the airways must be initiated. Continuous night pulse oximetry can be used for screening of the nigh time hypoxemia. Currently, it is not recommended to routinely monitor SaO_2 at home, more studies being required for this issue [11, 14, 16].

Blood gases or capnography allows the assessment and evaluation of the initial morning hypercapnia; then, it becomes permanent. Blood gases should be performed if $SaO_2 < 94\%$ and the patient do not have lung disease [16, 17]. In children with NMD, the use of capnography is preferred, a noninvasive method, in order to determine the transcutaneous CO_2, and to monitor the exchange of gases routinely [11, 14].

Polysomnography represents a diagnostical investigation option for respiratory disturbances during sleep and during alveolar hypoventilation in NMD and is the most pertinent indicator for proposing NIV [10, 21]. Polysomnography (**Figures 1** and **2**) is useful in nonambulant patients who cannot stand without any help and can be used for initiation and titration of the respiratory support, more specifically non-invasive ventilation. If polysomnography is not available, the cardiorespiratory polygraph is recommended, with a minimum of four channels: O_2 saturation, cardiac frequency, nasal flow, and chest movements during sleep [11, 14, 16].

A specific evaluation of respiratory muscle strength is the measurement of maximum inspiratory pressure (MIP), maximum expiratory pressure (MEP), and sniff nasal pressure (SNIP). In some patients, specifically in NMD with bulbar determination, some discrepancies are registered between the maximum inspiratory pressure (MIP) and sniff nasal pressure (SNIP). As a consequence of the discrepancies, it is recommended to do both tests, taking note to select the highest pressure [11, 16].

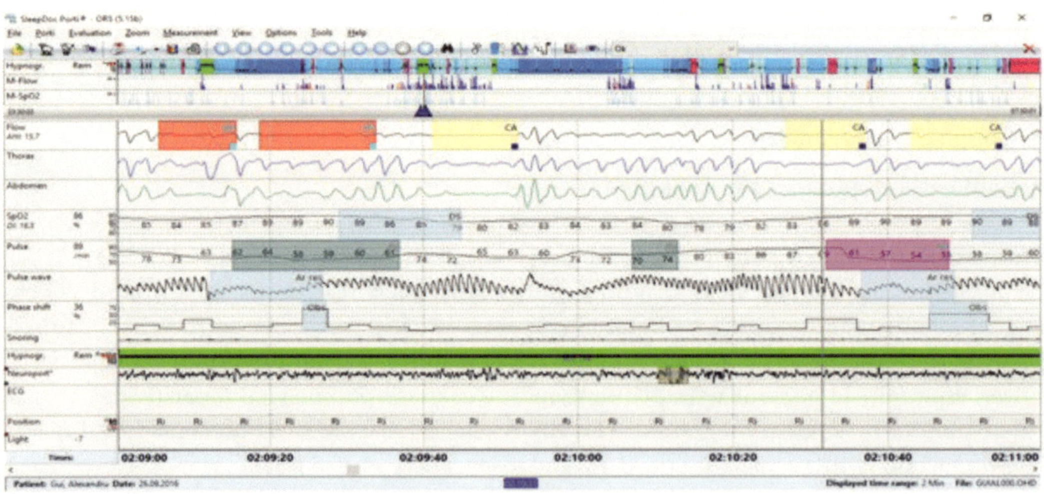

Figure 1. Polysomnography in 9 years old patient with Central Core Myopathy. Obstructive and central apnoea, AH1 = 15,7/hour of sleep, desaturation in O2 in REM sleep.

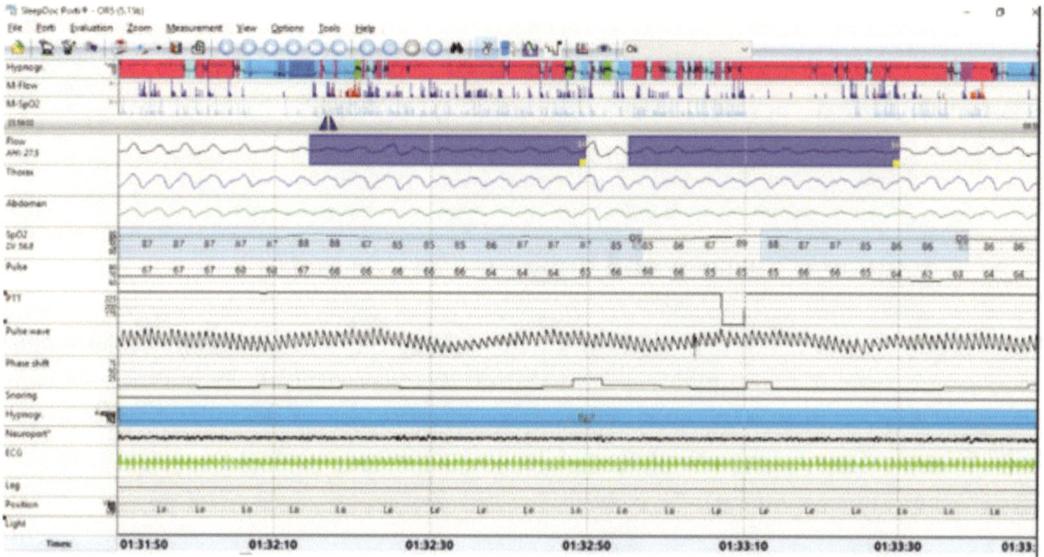

Figure 2. Polysomnography in a patient aged 45 years with ALS generalized form, spastic tetraplegia, pseudobulbar syndrome, syalorrhoea, eating difficulties, dyspnoea. Epoch with predominantly hypopneic flow, accompanied by desaturations in O_2, in stage N_2, morning PCO_2 = 51 mmHG.

5. Indications and contraindications for long-term NIV in NMD

The most frequent indications for NIV in NMD are:

- Amyotrophic lateral sclerosis (ALS)
- Duchenne's muscular dystrophy
- Becker's muscular dystrophy
- Steinert's muscular dystrophy
- Myasthenia gravis
- Spinal muscular atrophy [2, 7, 13, 15]

Depending on the natural evolution of neuromuscular disease to respiratory distress, NIV can be introduced to the management of the disease as soon as possible.

Contraindications for NIV in NMD:

- Facial burns/trauma/facial surgery or recent upper respiratory tract surgery
- Anatomical or functional obstruction
- Gastrointestinal or ileus bleeding

- Vomiting
- Hypersalivation
- Severe hypercapnia or severe respiratory acidosis (pH < 7.1)
- Without patient's consent for setting up NIV [2, 7, 15].

6. Neuromuscular diseases and long-term NIV: when?

There is plenty of evidence that precociously introducing NIV to the neuromuscular patient brings improvements in the quality of life and even prolongs survival. The question the clinician must ask is: when is the optimum moment for starting NIV with the neuromuscular patient?

NIV must be initiated when:

- The neuromuscular patient shows signs and symptoms of respiratory disturbances
- pCO_2 in the morning >45 mmHg
- FVC < 50% predicted value
- MIP or SNIP<60 mmHg
- Nocturnal SaO_2 < 88% for more than 5 min while under room air [1, 2, 14, 17].

Or

- FVC < 80% predicted value plus any symptoms or signs of respiratory impairment
- SNIP or MIP < 65 cm H_2O for men or 55 cm H_2O for women plus any symptoms or signs of respiratory impairment, particularly orthopnoea [17].

The classical indications to start NIV, when pCO_2 > 45 mmHg or when a patient has an exacerbation, as markers for respiratory failure could be too late. The history of neuromuscular diseases has a prolonged period of discrete symptoms of respiratory impairment, but with variable period of nocturnal hypoventilation. Performing polysomnography every year in a neuromuscular patient, as a routine method of disease monitoring, we can identify nocturnal hypoventilation very early and NIV could be started early [10]. Starting NIV earlier in the course of respiratory failure should be accompanied by a significant improvement in quality of life, and probably in prolonging life. There is no data for the moment to demonstrate this [10].

7. Introducing NIV in NMD, ventilator choices, interfaces

Non-invasive ventilation in NMD improved or corrected diurnal hypoxemia and hypercapnia, improved nocturnal hypoventilation and increases maximal respiratory pressures [7, 11, 14, 15, 22].

From the clinical point of view, NIV improved quality of life, control of symptoms of sleep related breathing, for example, headaches, sleep fragmentation, decreased daytime sleepiness, increased ability to perform daily activities, provide patients with sense of control and autonomy in advance stages, reduce hospitalizations and prolonged survival [1, 2, 3, 7].

Type of ventilators for long-term NIV:

- Pressure-support ventilator
- Volume-targeted ventilator: deliver known tidal volumes, but most machines have a limited capacity to correct leaks, leading to underventilation
- Hybrid mode ventilator: pressure-targeted volume-assured mod

Bi-level positive airway pressure ventilator (BiPAP), spontaneous/timed (S/T) mode is the most common type of pressure-support ventilator used for long-term NIV in NMD. There is a lack of study to compare different types of ventilators used for long-term NIV. But, pressure-targeted ventilators tend to be lighter and cheaper and also comfortable to the patient than volume-targeted ventilators [6, 11, 18].

Intelligent volume-assured pressure support (iVAPS) is a hybrid mode ventilator, providing constant automatic adjustment of pressure support (PS) to achieve a target ventilation determined by the patient's pathology [11, 18]. iVAPS demonstrated, in small studies, similar arterial

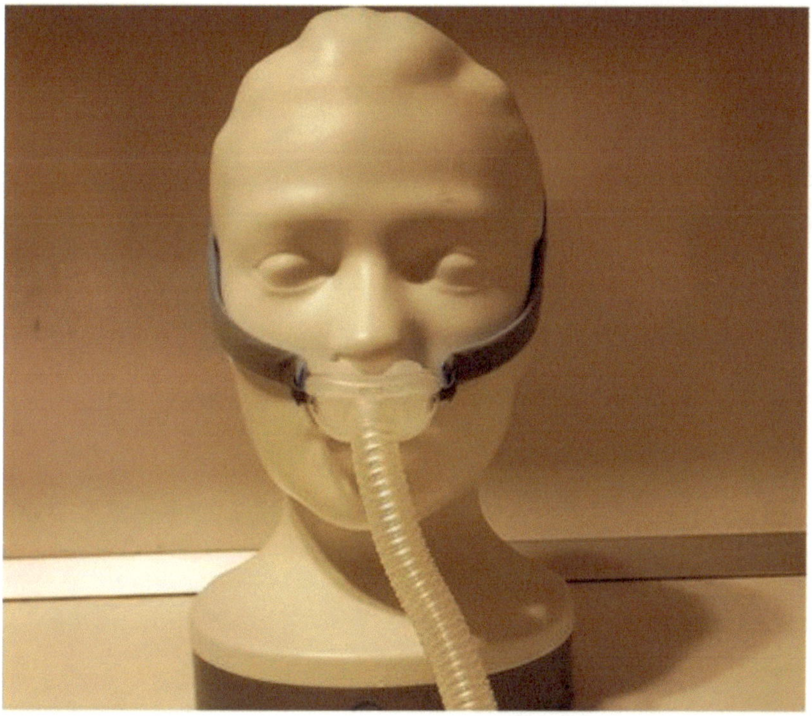

Figure 3. Choosing the interfaces: Pillow mask.

blood gases control to BiPAP, but iVAPS had higher overnight adherence, due to better patient-ventilator synchrony; there was no difference in outcome between ventilator modes for spirometry, respiratory muscle strength, sleep quality, arousals or O_2 desaturation index [11, 18].

7.1. Choosing the interfaces

Extremely important for good compliance to NIV is choosing the right interfaces. Nasal mask and pillow mask are best suited for cooperative patients that have a lower severity of the disease, or for children, needed low to moderate pressures only (< 20 cm H_2O). It also allows the patient to speak, drink, cough and clear his/her secretions while receiving the treatment. Nasal masks are more prone to leaks and the effectiveness is limited in patients with nasal obstructions, septal defects or other kind of deformities. Nasal and pillow mask are more comfortable for the patient than orofacial mask [11, 38, 39].

Orofacial mask, which encompass the mouth and nose are best suited for less cooperative patients who have more or less severe illnesses. It particularly fits patients who are mouth-breathing and edentulous and they are contraindicated in claustrophobic patients. Orofacial mask does not allow the patient to talk or eat and it is more uncomfortable for the patient than nasal or pillow mask [11, 38, 39].

Nasal mask, pillow mask and orofacial mask are illustrated in **Figures 3–5**.

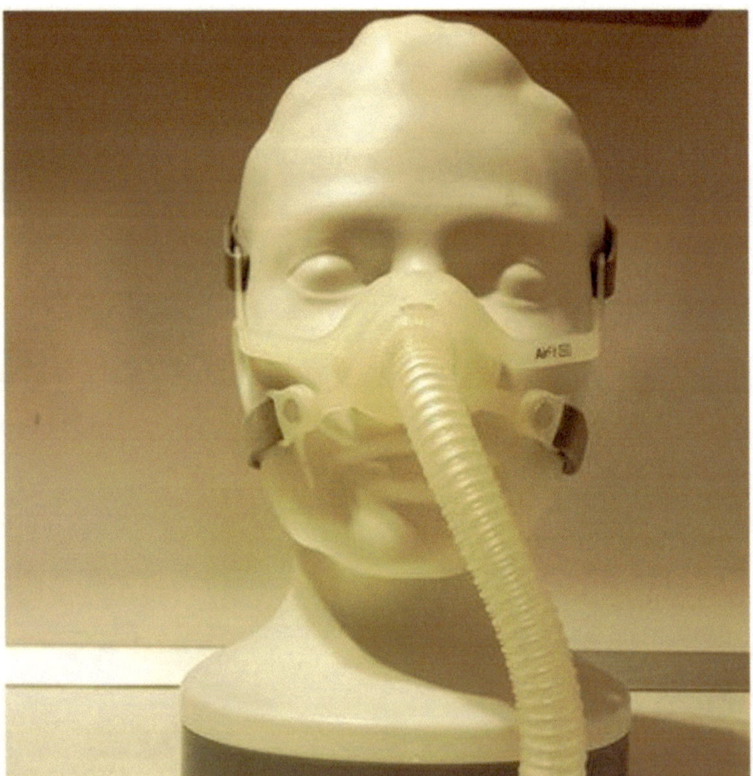

Figure 4. Choosing the interfaces: Nasal mask.

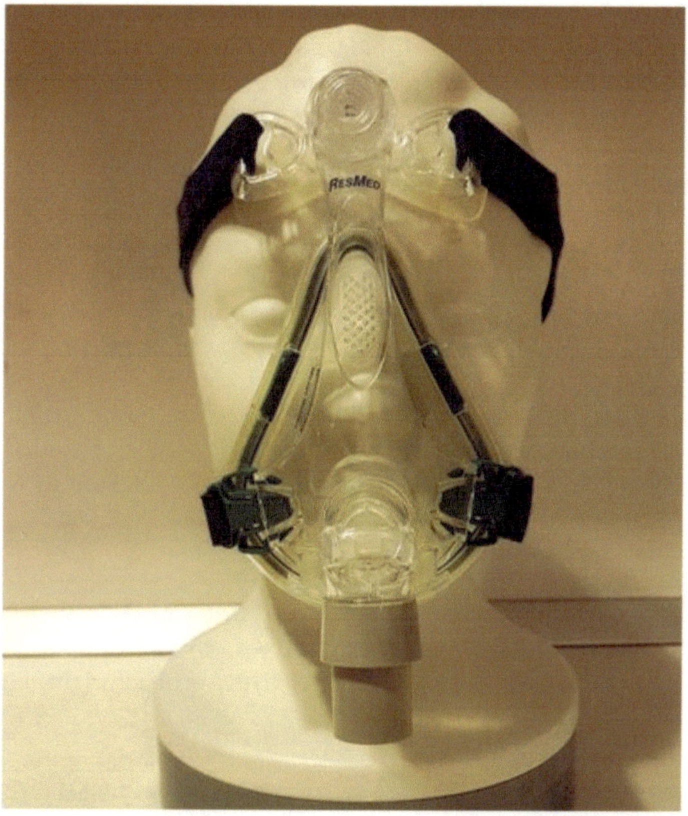

Figure 5. Choosing the interfaces: Orofacial mask.

7.1.1. Adverse effects and complications of NIV

The majority of adverse events of NIV are related to the mask: discomfort, skin rush, claustrophobia, nasal ulceration nasal congestion, eyes irritation, nasal or oral dryness. This mask related adverse events could be easily resolved by changing the interface and adding humidifier for the dryness of the mucosa.

Other NIV complications are aspiration pneumonia, pneumothorax or hypotension, with a low frequency < 5% [11, 38, 39].

8. Monitoring NIV in NMD

Effectiveness of NIV depended on a several factors: settings, interfaces, compliance and adherence of the patient to his ventilator. For obtaining a good compliance and adherence to NIV, monitoring NIV is crucial. The minimum requirement is a sleep study recording continuous oximetry, capnography or blood gases.

The frequency of monitoring NIV is depending of the cases; for new cases, monitoring is required to be done more often, every few weeks, until established that we obtained correction of nocturnal hypoventilation and blood gases. In stable cases on home-ventilation, with slowly progressive or non-progressive disease, annual assessment is sufficient [11, 38]. The new type of ventilators provided a compliance card, which permitted a minimum set of data to monitor: hours of usage, AHI index, leaks.

8.1. Using ultrasound to monitor NIV in NMD

One of the main causes of morbidity and mortality in patients with neuromuscular diseases (NMD) is respiratory failure. The diaphragm acts as the main respiratory muscle during inspiration and accounts for 70% of the inspired air volume during regular breathing [19]. The diaphragm function can indirectly be analyzed by techniques such as fluoroscopy and chest radiography, which are non-specific and also ionizing exams [23]. Ultrasound (US) as a non-invasive, radiation-free imaging tool, allows an accurate, reproducible and safe assessment of diaphragm anatomy and function at the bedside [24–27]. Ultrasound has been shown to be similar in accuracy to most other imaging modalities for diaphragm assessment [28].

8.1.1. Technique of diaphragmatic ultrasound (US) assessment

With ultrasound, the diaphragm is typically identified by its deep location, curved shape and muscular echo-structure. Longitudinally it has a mixed echogenic appearance, consisting of hypo echoic (dark) muscle fibers separated by two hyper echoic (bright) layers: peritoneum and pleura (**Figure 6**).

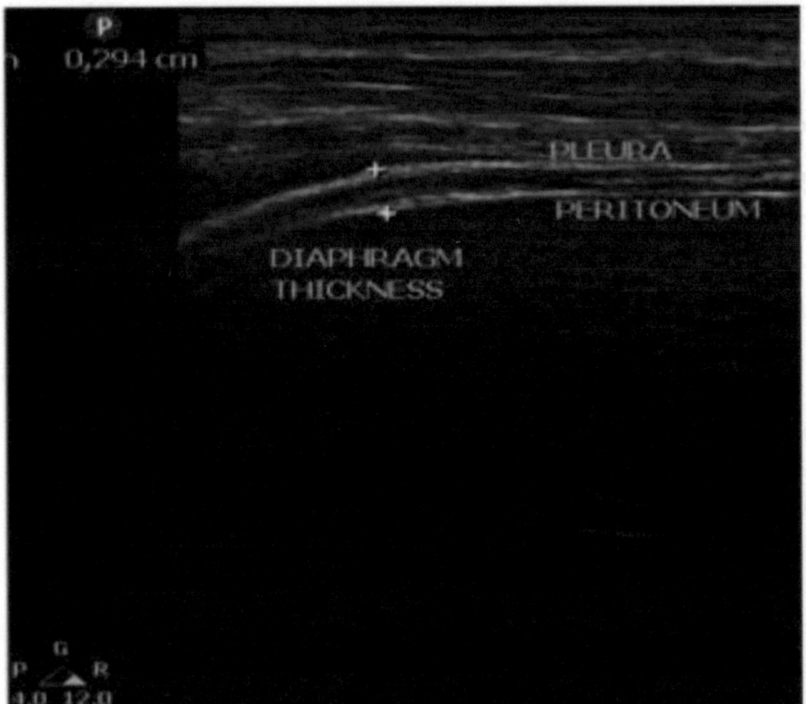

Figure 6. Normal US appearance and thickness of the diaphragm.

Patients are typically examined during spontaneous respiration to help identify the diaphragm moving. The supine position of the patient is preferred, because there is less overall variability, less side-to-side variability, and greater reproducibility [29]. Also, it could identify any paradoxical movement.

The right diaphragm can be visualized through the liver window. Visualization of the left diaphragm could be sometimes more difficult because of the smaller window of the spleen.

Classically, there are two methods to evaluate the diaphragm: the analyses of the movement of diaphragmatic dome using the M mode and the measurement of diaphragmatic thickness and the thickening during inspiration in the area of apposition using the B mode.

The anterior subcostal view is preferred for evaluation of diaphragm excursion. It requires a lower frequency, ideally curvilinear, transducer (2–6 MHz) placed between the mid-clavicular and anterior axillary lines (**Figure 7**), so that the ultrasound beam could reach the posterior third of the diaphragm. B mode is used to visualize the diaphragm moving toward or away from the transducer. Imaging is then changed to M mode with the line of sight positioned in order to obtain maximum excursion (**Figure 8**). Either dome of the diaphragm can be evaluated using the liver and spleen window and the amplitude of excursion can be measured on M mode, and diaphragm velocity can be calculated (**Figure 8**).

For an intercostal view, a higher frequency linear array transducer (7–18 MHz) is placed at the anterior axillary line, with the transducer positioned to obtain a sagittal image at the intercostal space between the 7th and 8th, or 8th and 9th ribs (**Figure 9**). The zone of apposition is assessed for measurement of the diaphragm thickness and echogenicity.

8.1.2. Measurements

Diaphragm thickness is measured at the zone of apposition during inspiration or expiration using the intercostal approach. The average thickness of the diaphragm is 0.22–0.28 cm in healthy volunteers [30]. Diaphragm thickness less than 0.2 cm, measured at the end of expiration, have been proposed as the cut-off to define diaphragm atrophy [31].

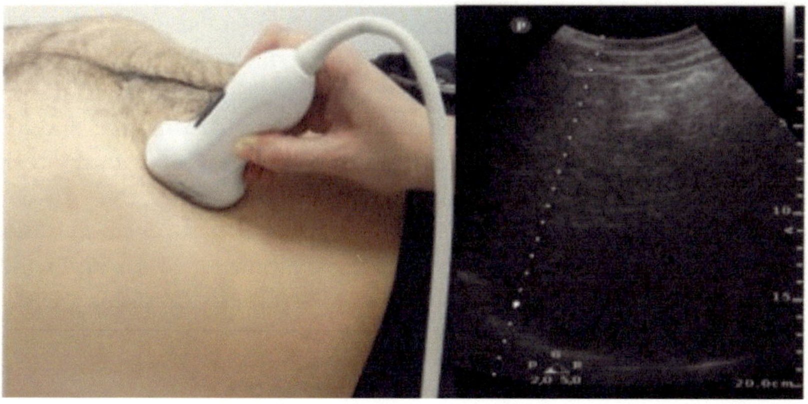

Figure 7. Diaphragm assessment in anterior subcostal view.

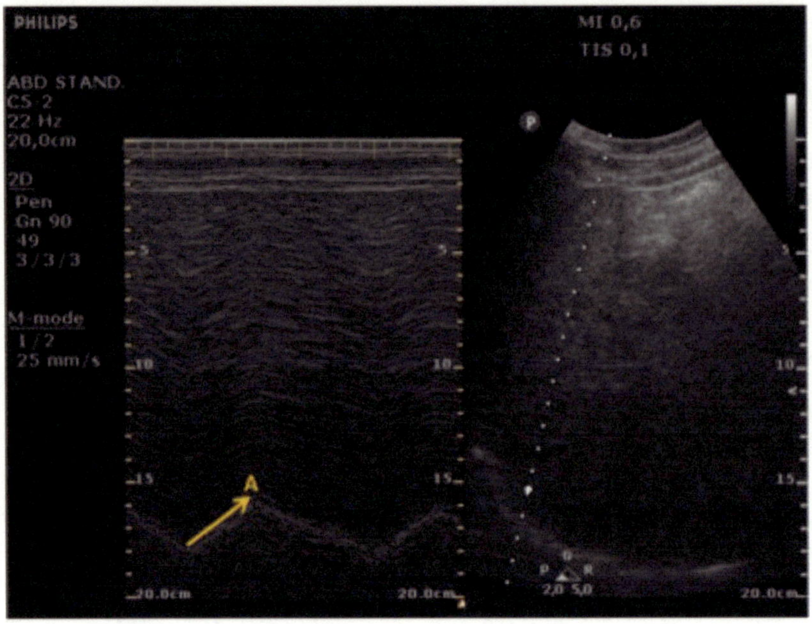

Figure 8. Assessment of diaphragm movement in M mode and 2D mode (A-wave amplitude).

Muscle fibers shorten with contraction and cause muscle thickening. A chronically paralyzed diaphragm is thin, atrophic, and does not thicken during inspiration. The measurement of thickness alone may miss an acutely paralyzed diaphragm with normal thickness or could incorrectly identify atrophy in a low weight individual with a healthy, yet thin, diaphragm. Therefore, the degree of diaphragm thickening has been proposed to be more sensitive than measurement of thickness alone [32]. Thickening fraction (TF) was calculated as: [thickness at end-inspiration (TEI)–thickness at end-expiration (TEE)]/TEE and expressed as a percentage (TEI thickness at end-inspiration; TEE thickness at end-expiration). Diaphragm thickening of less than 20% is proposed to be consistent with paralysis [32].

Diaphragm movement is recorded using the M mode assessment of the dome in the anterior subcostal view. The diaphragm is seen as a single thick echogenic line, and its movements with respiration can be plotted against a time curve. Measurement of the amplitude of excursion can be used to compare movement of the two hemi-diaphragms and for follow-up of diaphragmatic function (**Figure 8**). The normal range of motion from the resting expiratory position to full inspiration in adults has been reported to range from 1.9 cm in normal breathing to 9 cm in deep breathing [33]. Excursion greater than 2.5 cm in adults has been proposed as a cut-off for excluding severe diaphragm dysfunction [34]. Diaphragm weakness is indicated by less than normal amplitude of excursion on deep breathing with or without paradoxical motion on sniffing. Some variations are mentioned related to sex, age, weight or height.

http://dx.doi.org/10.5772/intechopen.77173

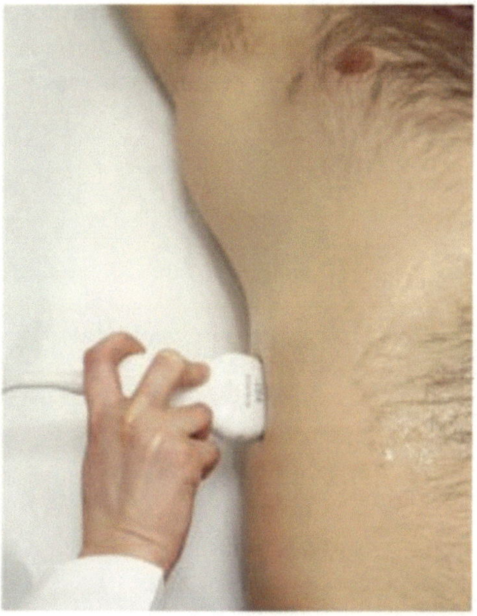

Figure 9. Diaphragm assessment in intercostal view, using a high frequency linear probe.

8.1.3. Clinical application

Mechanical ventilation is associated with decreased muscle weight and alterations in contractile properties of the diaphragm within 48 h of intubation [35]. Diaphragm dysfunction may contribute to weaning failure, even in patients with no obvious reason to suspect phrenic nerve or diaphragm pathology. Decreased diaphragm excursion on M-mode ultrasound has been shown to predict weaning failure, with a 1.4 cm cut-off for the right hemidiaphragm and 1.2 cm for the left hemidiaphragm [36].

In critically ill patients under non-invasive ventilation, the diaphragm thickness and the thickening fraction (TF) are decreased as the level of pressure support increased (5, 10, 15 cm H_2O). The measurements done in the zone of apposition during tidal ventilation showed that, during NIV, thickening of the diaphragm is due to muscle effort and not due to increase in pulmonary volume induced by ventilation [37].

TF could be used in the ICU setting to assess diaphragmatic function and could contribute to respiratory workload in various situations, including ventilator-induced diaphragmatic dysfunction and ICU-acquired paresis [32].

9. Conclusions

Non-invasive ventilation in neuromuscular diseases should be introduced earlier in the evolution of respiratory failure, for obtaining maximum benefit for the quality of life, control of symptoms, increased ability to perform daily activities, reduce hospitalizations and prolonged survival. Choosing the ventilator, the most appropriate interface, the ventilation mode, and periodic monitoring of the NIV is essential in obtaining success.

Abbreviations

ALS	Amyotrophic lateral sclerosis
BiPAP	bi-level positive airway pressure ventilator
DMD	Duchenne muscular dystrophy
FVC	forced vital capacity
iVAPS	intelligent volume-assured pressure support
NMD	neuromuscular disease
NIV	non-invasive ventilation
pCO_2	arterial pressure of CO_2
PS	pressure support
REM	rapid eyes movement sleep
S/T	spontaneous/timed
SNIP	sniff nasal pressure
US	ultrasound
TF	thickening fraction
MIP	maximum inspiratory pressure
MEP	maximum expiratory pressure

Author details

Lavinia Davidescu[1], Diana Manolescu[2*], Ruxandra Ulmeanu[3] and Cristian Oancea[2]

*Address all correspondence to: dr.dianamanolescu@gmail.com

1 Faculty of Medicine, University of Medicine Oradea, Romania

2 Faculty of Medicine, University of Medicine "Victor Babes" Timisoara, Romania

3 Marius Nasta Institute, Faculty of Medicine, University of Medicine Oradea, Bucuresti, Romania

References

[1] Shneerson JM, Simonds AK. Non-invasive ventilation for chest wall and neuromuscular disorders. European Respiratory Journal. 2002;**20**:480-487. DOI: 10.1183/09031936.02.00404002

[2] Simonds AK. Chronic NIV in hereditary neuromuscular disorders, ERS Practical Handbook of Noninvasive ventilation, In: Paolo Palange, Anita K, Simonds, editors. ERS Book. 2015. pp. 163-175. DOI: 10.1183/9781849840415-hba02

[3] Fauroux B. ERS School Course-NIV in neuromuscular diseases. Hanover 2012. Available from: http://www.ers-education.org/events/courses/noninvasive-positive-pressure-ventilation,-hanover-2012.aspx [Accessed: March 05, 2018]

[4] Pinto S et al. Predicting respiratory insufficiency in ALS. Clinical Neurophysiology. 2009; **120**(5):941-946. Epub 2009 Apr 1

[5] Pinto AC, Evangelista T, Carvalho M, Alves MA, Sales Luis ML. Respiratory assistance with a non-invasive ventilator (BiPAP) in MND/ALS patients: Survival rates in a controlled trial. Journal of the Neurological Sciences. 1995;**129**(Suppl):19-26

[6] Ambrosino N, Carpenè N, Gherardi M. Chronic respiratory care for neuromuscular diseases in adults. European Respiratory Journal. Aug 2009;**34**(2):444-451. DOI: 10.1183/09031936.00182208

[7] Lisboa C, Díaz O, Fadic R. Noninvasive mechanical ventilation in patients with neuromuscular diseases and in patients with chest restriction. Archivos de Bronconeumología. 2003;**39**:314-320 Vol. 39 Num. 7

[8] Lo Mauro A, Aliverti A. Physiology of respiratory disturbances in muscular dystrophies. Breathe. 2016;**12**(4):318-327. DOI: 10.1183/20734735.012716

[9] Hutchinson D, Whyte K. Neuromuscular diseases and respiratory failure. Practical neurology. 2008;**8**:229-237. DOI: 10.1136/pn.2008.152611

[10] Fauroux B, Lofaso F. Non-invasive mechanical ventilation: When to start for what benefit? Thorax. 2005;**60**:979-980

[11] Hull J, Aniapravan R, Chan E, et al. British Thoracic Society guideline for respiratory management of children with neuromuscular weakness. Thorax. 2012;**67**:i1-i40

[12] Goncalves MR, Bach JR. Mechanical insufflation-exsufflation improves outcomes for neuromuscular disease patients with respiratory tract infections: A step in rightdirection. American Journal of Physical Medicine & Rehabilitation. 2005;**84**:89-91

[13] Hill NS. Neuromuscular disease in respiratory and critical care medicine. Respiratory Care. 2006;**51**(9):1065-1071

[14] Birnkrant D et al. Diagnosis and management of Duchene muscular distrophy part 2: Respiratory, cardiac, bone health and ortopaedic management. The Lancet Neurology. April 2018;**17**(4):347-361. DOI: 10.1016/S1474-4422(18)30025-5

[15] Janssens JP. Indications in long term NIV in chronic respiratory failure-ERS Course NIV, Hanover, 2017. Available from: http://www.erseducation.org/events/courses/noninvasive-ventilation-basic-concepts,-hanover-2017.aspx [Accessed: March 01, 2018]

[16] Perez T. Amyotrophic lateral sclerosis (ALS): Evaluation of respiratory function. Revue Neurologique (Paris). 2006 Jun;**162**: Spec No 2:4S188-4S194

[17] Nice Guideline—Motor neurone disease: Assessment and management, 2016. Available from: https://www.nice.org.uk/guidance/ng42 [Accessed: February 28, 2018]

[18] Kelly JL, Jaye J, Pickersgill RE, Simonds AK. Randomized trial of 'intelligent' autotitrating ventilation versus standard pressure support non-invasive ventilation: Impact on adherence and physiological outcomes. Respirology. 2014;**9**(4):596-603. https://doi.org/10.1111/resp.1226

[19] Mead J, Loring SH. Analysis of volume displacement and length changes of the diaphragm during breathing. Journal of Applied Physiology: Respiratory, Environmental and Exercise Physiology. 1982;**53**(3):750-755

[20] D'Angelo MG, Romei M, Lo Mauro A, et al. Respiratory pattern in an adult population of dystrophic patients. Journal of the Neurological Sciences. 2011;**306**:54-61

[21] Kang PB, Morrison L, Iannaccone ST, et al. Evidence-based guideline summary: Evaluation, diagnosis, and management of congenital muscular dystrophy. Neurology. 2015;**84**:1369-1378

[22] Perrin C, Unterborn JN, Ambrosio CD, et al. Pulmonary complications of chronic neuromuscular diseases and their management. Muscle & Nerve. 2004;**29**:5-27

[23] Chavhan GB, Babyn PS, Cohen RA, Langer JC. Multimodality imaging of the pediatric diaphragm: Anatomy and pathologic conditions. Radiographics. 2010;**30**(7):1797-1817

[24] Ueki J, De Bruin PF, Pride NB. In vivo assessment of diaphragm contraction by ultrasound in normal subjects. Thorax. 1995;**50**(11):1157-1161

[25] Kantarci F, Mihmanli I, Demirel MK, Harmanci K, Akman C, Aydogan F, Mihmanli A, Uysal O. Normal diaphragmatic motion and the effects of body composition: Determination with M-mode sonography. Journal of Ultrasound in Medicine. 2004;**23**(2):255-260

[26] Cohn D, Benditt JO, Eveloff S, FD MC. Diaphragm thickening during inspiration. Journal of Applied Physiology. 1997;**83**(1):291-296

[27] Boon AJ, Harper CJ, Ghahfarokhi LS, Strommen JA, Watson JC, Sorenson EJ. Two-dimensional ultrasound imaging of the diaphragm: Quantitative values in normal subjects. Muscle & Nerve. 2013;**47**(6):884-889

[28] Houston JG, Fleet M, Cowan MD, McMillan NC. Comparison of ultrasound with fluoroscopy in the assessment of suspected hemidiaphragmatic movement abnormality. Clinical Radiology. 1995 Feb;**50**(2):95-98

[29] Gerscovich EO, Cronan M, McGahan JP, Jain K, Jones CD, McDonald C. Ultrasonographic evaluation of diaphragmatic motion. Journal of Ultrasound in Medicine. 2001 Jun;**20**(6):597-604

[30] Wait JL, Nahormek PA, Yost WT, Rochester DP. Diaphragmatic thickness-lung volume relationship in vivo. Journal of Applied Physiology. 1989 Oct;**67**(4):1560-1568

[31] Gottesman E, McCool FD. Ultrasound evaluation of the paralyzed diaphragm. American Journal of Respiratory and Critical Care Medicine. 1997 May;**155**(5):1570-1574

[32] Summerhill EM, El-Sameed YA, Glidden TJ, McCool FD. Monitoring recovery from diaphragm paralysis with ultrasound. Chest. 2008 Mar;**133**(3):737-743

[33] Ayoub J, Cohendy R, Dauzat M, Targhetta R, De la Coussaye JE, Bourgeois JM, Ramonatxo M, Prefaut C, Pourcelot L. Non-invasive quantification of diaphragm kinetics using m-mode sonography. Canadian Journal of Anaesthesia. 1997 Jul;**44**(7):739-744

[34] Lerolle N, Guerot E, Dimassi S, Zegdi R, Faisy C, Fagon JY, Diehl JL. Ultrasonographic diagnostic criterion for severe diaphragmatic dysfunction after cardiac surgery. Chest. 2009 Feb;**135**(2):401-407

[35] Capdevila X, Lopez S, Bernard N, Rabischong E, Ramonatxo M, Martinazzo G, Prefaut C. Effects of controlled mechanical ventilation on respiratory muscle contractile properties in rabbits. Intensive Care Medicine. 2003 Jan;**29**(1):103-110

[36] Kim WY, Suh HJ, Hong SB, Koh Y, Lim CM. Diaphragm dysfunction assessed by ultrasonography: Influence on weaning from mechanical ventilation. Critical Care Medicine. 2011 Dec;**39**(12):2627-2630

[37] Vivier E, Mekontso Dessap A, Dimassi S, Vargas F, Lyazidi A, Thille WA, Brochard L. Diaphragm ultrasonography to estimate the work of breathing during non-invasive ventilation. Intensive Care Medicine. 2012;**38**:796-803

[38] Hasan A. Understanding mechanical ventilation: A Practical Handbook, 2nd ed.; London: Springer; 2010;**13**:420. DOI: 10.1007/978-1-84882-869-8

[39] Köhnlein T. Interfaces for noninvasive ventilation, in ERS Course Non-invasive ventilation, Hannover, 2012. Available from: http://www.ers-education.org/events/courses/noninvasive-positive-pressure-ventilation,-hanover-2012.aspx [Accessed: February 28, 2018]

Chapter 4

Noninvasive Monitoring of Manual Ventilation during Out-of-Hospital Cardiopulmonary Resuscitation

Andoni Elola, Erik Alonso, Elisabete Aramendi and Unai Irusta

Additional information is available at the end of the chapter

http://dx.doi.org/10.5772/intechopen.77172

Abstract

Cardiopulmonary resuscitation (CPR) consisting of chest compressions and assisted ventilation is crucial to treat out-of-hospital cardiac arrest (OHCA). It is well reported that quality of manual ventilations, in terms of rate and volume, is suboptimal, with a high incidence of hyperventilation, which is linked to poor outcomes. The lack of a noninvasive technology to monitor ventilations during out-of-hospital CPR precludes feedback on ventilations to the rescuer, and it handicaps the evaluation of the effect of ventilations on the outcome of the patient. This chapter addresses the possibilities and challenges of monitoring the quality of manual ventilations in current defibrillators. Methods are proposed to monitor ventilations based on the thoracic impedance and the capnogram. These methods can be integrated in defibrillators used in both basic and advanced life support. The algorithms are described, and the accuracy of the methods to monitor the ventilation rate and the quality metrics of the ventilations is reported using real OHCA episodes. The accuracy and limitations of the methods as well as the implications of integrating them in the treatment of patients in cardiac arrest are discussed.

Keywords: manual ventilation, cardiopulmonary resuscitation, out-of-hospital cardiac arrest, thoracic impedance, capnogram

1. Introduction

Sudden cardiac arrest is the sudden cessation of effective blood circulation due to heart failure. If not treated promptly, cardiac arrest can lead to sudden cardiac death within minutes [1]. Sudden cardiac death is one of the leading causes of death in the industrialized world [2, 3].

Although the overall incidence depends on the definition and inclusion criteria applied by each study, it is documented that it ranges from 150,000 to 530,000 person-year in the United States, and about 275,000 in Europe [1, 2, 4].

Most cardiac arrest occur in the out-of-hospital setting [5]. There are two levels of treatment for out-of-hospital cardiac arrest (OHCA), basic life support delivered by emergency medical technicians and advanced life support (ALS) with the intervention of clinicians. Despite important progress in epidemiology, profiling and treatment of OHCA in the last decades, the survival rates to hospital discharge are dismally low, with rates between 8.4 and 10.7% [2, 6].

In OHCA, the first minutes are crucial as the chances of the patient to survive decrease about 10% per minute [7]. The chain of survival defines the key steps to treat a person in cardiac arrest. Two of the most important links of the chain are early defibrillation and early cardiopulmonary resuscitation (CPR). Defibrillation is delivered either by an automated external defibrillator (AED) or by more advanced monitor defibrillators used by ALS clinicians. The objective of CPR is to maintain a minimum oxygenated blood flow to the heart and brain until advanced care is available.

Quality of CPR is a key factor for the survival of OHCA patients. The 2015 resuscitation guidelines recommend that chest compression are provided with a rate of at least 100 compressions per minute and a depth of 5 cm [8]. During CPR, two ventilations may be given between series of chest compressions before intubation. Lay rescuers should open the airway using a head-tilt-chin-lift maneuver and blow steadily into the mouth while watching for the chest to rise, as shown in **Figure 1** [9]. The time taken to give a ventilation should be around 1 s, with no more than 5 s for two ventilations. After intubation, the resuscitation guidelines recommend CPR including continuous bag-mask ventilation with and without supplementary oxygen, as shown in **Figure 2**. The recommended ventilation rate is about 1 breath every 5–6 s, or about 10–12 breaths per minute [11]. However excessive ventilation, either by rate or tidal volume is

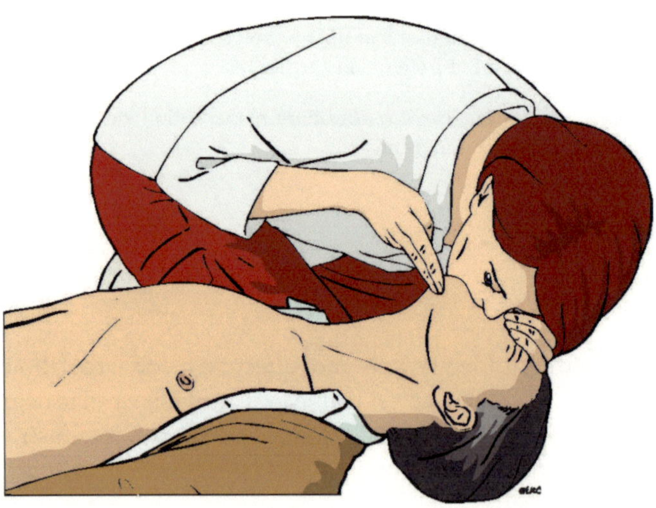

Figure 1. Head-tilt-chin-lift maneuver to provide ventilations. Extracted from [9].

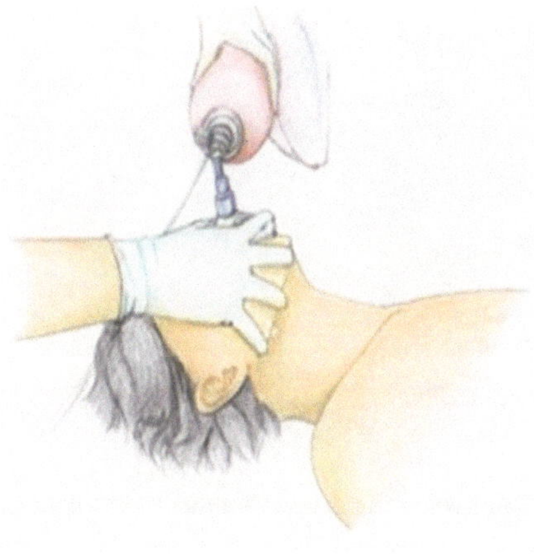

Figure 2. Bag-mask ventilation. Extracted from [10].

common during resuscitation [12–16]. Several analyses on OHCA episodes report rates ranging from moderate (14 min^{-1}) to severe (>20 min^{-1}) hyperventilation.

The negative effect of hyperventilation during CPR is well known: it increases intrathoracic pressures, reshapes the oxygen dissociation curve (increasing oxygen affinity) and behaves as a cerebral vasoconstrictor [17, 18]. Many studies have also proven that it contributes to a lower coronary perfusion pressure and to hemodynamic deterioration in animals [19, 20]. All these factors decrease the probability of survival of a patient in cardiac arrest, so the monitoring and evaluation of ventilation during CPR.

The real-time monitoring of the instantaneous ventilation rate during OHCA would enable feedback to the rescuers, so they could adhere to current guidelines. Furthermore, retrospective evaluation of the ventilation rates may help in debriefing to improve the quality of CPR provided by emergency medical services. Unfortunately, no commercial systems are available for BLS or ALS defibrillation equipment that give real-time feedback to the providers, and no automatic methods are available for debriefing on the quality of ventilation. Several quality metrics have been proposed to monitor quality of ventilations in OHCA [21], such as the mean value of ventilations delivered per minute and the fraction of minutes with hyperventilation (FMH), that is ventilation rates above 15 min^{-1}.

The automated computation of those ventilation quality values requires ventilation detection algorithms based on signal processing of the biomedical signals recorded by commercial equipment. Nowadays, equipment to monitor gas exchange during ventilations is not routinely used in OHCA, in contrast to the ubiquitous mechanical ventilators used in-hospital. In the BLS scenario, the biomedical signals recorded by AEDs through the defibrillation pads (see **Figure 3**) are most frequently the electrocardiogram (ECG) and the thoracic impedance (TI). Ventilations are visible in the TI as fluctuations in the waveform with every insufflation of oxygen into the chest of the patient. For more advanced monitor-defibrillators, as the ones used by medical experts in ALS, additional modules like the capnogram are available. Capnography monitors the partial pressure of the CO_2 in the respiratory gasses, and reflects high concentration during the exhalation phase of every ventilation.

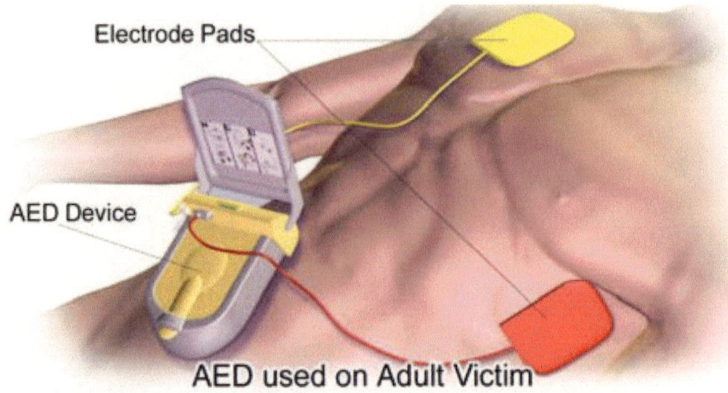

Figure 3. Automated external defibrillator with electrode pads attached to a patient.

In this chapter, the feasibility of monitoring the ventilation rate is analyzed using first the TI and then the capnogram. Automatic methods to detect ventilations are described, and their accuracy reported with OHCA datasets. The performance of the algorithms is reported in terms of sensitivity (SE), the percentage of correctly detected ventilations, and positive predictive value (PPV), the percentage of detected ventilations that are true ventilations. The validity of those methods to monitor the instantaneous ventilation rate and to evaluate the quality of ventilation is also analyzed. Finally, this chapter concludes with a discussion of several key points to be considered before these methods could be integrated into commercial equipment.

2. Thoracic impedance for ventilation monitoring

The TI is measured though the defibrillation pads of a defibrillator attached to the chest of the patient in the anterolateral position, as shown in **Figure 3**. A high frequency excitation current (20–100 kHz at 1–5 mA) is applied through the pads and the resulting surface potential measured to compute the impedance by applying Ohm's law. The TI may show different components:

- *Baseline component*: a baseline impedance value of 50–120 Ω depending on the position of the pads and on the patient's sex, chest size and body mass [22].
- *Chest compression component*: chest compressions cause variations in the cross-sectional area of the chest [23] and mechanical disturbances in the defibrillation pads that are reflected in the TI as fluctuations of amplitudes between 0.15 Ω and several ohms [24, 25].
- *Ventilation component*: ventilations produce variations in the cross-sectional area of the thorax [23]. Inflation of the lungs causes an increase in impedance because air is a poor conductor of electric current [25]. The TI shows a fluctuation from 0.1 Ω to 8 Ω with each ventilation [26, 27].
- *Circulation component*: the impedance shows a small fluctuation (<100 mΩ) with each effective heartbeat [26, 28, 29].
- *Additional noise and artifacts*: other noise and artifacts due to movement, electrode-skin contact, and so on can be present in the impedance [30].

http://dx.doi.org/10.5772/intechopen.77172

All these components can be observed in **Figure 4**. From top to bottom, the ECG, TI, the compression depth (CD) of the chest compressions and the capnography are depicted. The TI shows a baseline around 105 Ω and fluctuations due to chest compressions (around 1 Ω), ventilations (0.5–1 Ω), and circulation (0.1 Ω). There is a perfect match between (1) compressions in the CD signal and fluctuations due to compressions in the TI signal, (2) the capnogram and fluctuations due to ventilations in the TI, and (3) effective heartbeats in the ECG and the circulation component in the TI. Two ventilations are visible in the TI, the fluctuations around 14 and 18 s, which correlate with increases of the CO_2 expired in the capnogram.

The TI has become a very useful signal in an OHCA in the last two decades and it is recorded by every commercial defibrillator, either AED or monitor/defibrillator. In 2002, Pellis et al. first suggested that ventilations (respirations) cause measurable fluctuations in the TI signal [27]. In an experiment with anesthetized male pigs, they found out that TI measurement at frequencies between 0.1 and 2 Hz showed fluctuations that were time coincident with the ventilations in the capnography signal.

Later in 2006, Losert et al. analyzed the feasibility of monitoring the ventilation characteristics during CPR using the TI signal acquired by the defibrillation pads of an AED [26]. They analyzed the correlation between the amplitude of the TI fluctuation due to ventilation and the tidal volume (400–1000 mL) given by a ventilator. They concluded that the TI

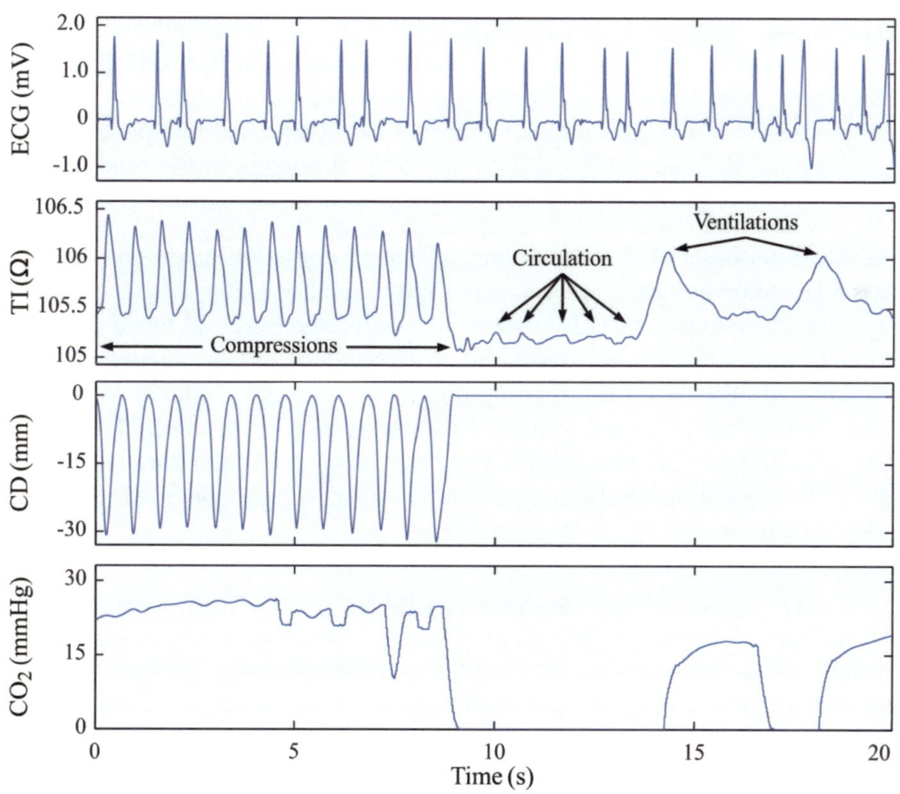

Figure 4. From top to bottom, the ECG, TI, CD and capnography signals are represented. Two ventilations are visible in the TI around 14 and 18 s.

allows to compute ventilation rates, inspiration and expiration times, but the amplitude of the TI fluctuation was not valid for exact tidal volume estimation. More recently, Roberts et al. also investigated the relationship between tidal volume and TI amplitude fluctuations but in mechanically ventilated children and using the TI acquired for two different placements of the defibrillation pads, anterior-apical and anterior-posterior positions [31]. The ventilations in the TI were detected as fluctuations above 0.4 Ω. The study concluded that although the linearity between tidal volume and TI fluctuation was high for each individual, it was not feasible to derive the exact tidal volume from the TI fluctuation for the pediatric population as a whole. The study also showed that the TI acquired via defibrillation pads could be used to accurately detect ventilations if delivered according to the guidelines (7–10 ml/kg tidal volume), with no significant differences between pad positions for ventilation detection. Nevertheless, for smaller volumes (<7 ml/kg), the sensitivity for ventilation detection decreased, suggesting that shallow ventilations during CPR might not be detected in the TI.

These evidences motivated Risdal et al. to propose a ventilation detector during CPR based on the TI signal [32]. After a preprocessing stage, the fluctuations in the TI due to chest compressions were suppressed using an adaptive filtering scheme [33]. The ventilation detector was based on a neural network classifier. The classifier decided whether each TI segment (1.4 s) analyzed was an expiration onset (maximum peak of the fluctuation in the TI) in the basis of waveform features extracted from the analyzed segment. This was a novel and complex approach to detect ventilations with excellent performance (SE/PPV of 90.4%/95.5%). However, ventilations were manually annotated in the TI signal and used as gold standard to evaluate the performance of the ventilation detector. Therefore, still there was the need for a more reliable validation using a robust independent gold standard. Furthermore, the complexity and computational burden of the method limited its application.

More recently, Edelson et al. developed two different ventilation detection algorithms, one based on the TI and other based on the capnography signal [34]. They hypothesized that capnography would be superior to TI for measuring ventilation rate, and that a combined algorithm would be more accurate than one based on a single signal. They obtained slightly better results in terms of SE/PPV for the capnography-based detector: 78%/87% for the TI-based detector, and 82%/91% for the capnography-based detector. As hypothesized the combination of both algorithms showed better performance. The lack of a gold standard (spirometry, flow or volume of the ventilations) independent of the signals used to develop the detectors might have affected the results.

2.1. An automated ventilation detector based on the TI

In this section, we present a study carried out to overcome the main limitations of the works described earlier and to cast some light on the reliability and accuracy of the TI to compute ventilation metrics. The study is aimed at (1) developing a simple ventilation detector based on the TI that might be incorporated into current commercial defibrillators; and (2) computing the CPR quality metrics related to ventilations in order to evaluate their accuracy against a robust gold standard.

The dataset used to carry out the study consisted of OHCA episodes recorded through the Philips MRx monitor/defibrillator between 2006 and 2009 by the Tualatin Valley Fire and Rescue in Portland, OR, USA. Each episode contained concurrent TI and capnography signals for at least 30 min. The capnogram was considered the gold standard for the instants of ventilations which were manually and independently annotated by three experienced biomedical engineers. Intervals where the ventilation pattern was not clearly recognizable were excluded from the analysis. A total of 2575 min were analyzed, which included 17,586 ventilations. Episodes were randomly allocated to training and test sets, 32 and 31 episodes respectively. **Figure 5** shows an epoch of an episode included in the dataset of the study where capnography and TI signals are depicted, and the instants of ventilations are marked as black dotted lines on the capnogram.

The ventilation detector was developed using the training set and consisted of three different stages. First, a preprocessing stage where the TI was low-pass filtered at a cutoff frequency of 0.6 Hz to suppress fluctuations due to chest compressions as well as high frequency noise. In a second stage, the preprocessed TI signal, pTI, was analyzed to detect the local maxima and minima. Each local maximum and minimum were characterized by its time of occurrence, t_{max_i} or t_{min_i}, and amplitude, Z_{max_i} or Z_{min_i}, respectively as shown in **Figure 6**.

Each detected local maximum was a potential ventilation. To decide whether a maximum corresponded to a ventilation, the inflation amplitude ($A = Z_{max_i} - Z_{min_i}$) and inflation time ($d = t_{max_i} - t_{min_i}$) were first computed. Then, in the third stage, a decision algorithm decided if a local maximum was a ventilation based on A and d. Three were the requirements for a potential ventilation to be classified as ventilation. The value of d should exceed a minimum static threshold ($d_{min} = 0.5$ s); the inflation amplitude, A, should be above a dynamic threshold (Th_v) that represents the weighted average of the minimum amplitude of the last 17 ventilations, and finally, the time interval between the actual fluctuation and last detected ventilation should exceed a refractory period ($T_{ref} = 1.4$ s).

This ventilation detector was used to detect the instants of ventilations, and these instants were used to compute the instantaneous ventilation rate, which is reported every 15 s as the ventilation rate provided in the last minute. The global quality metrics of every episode

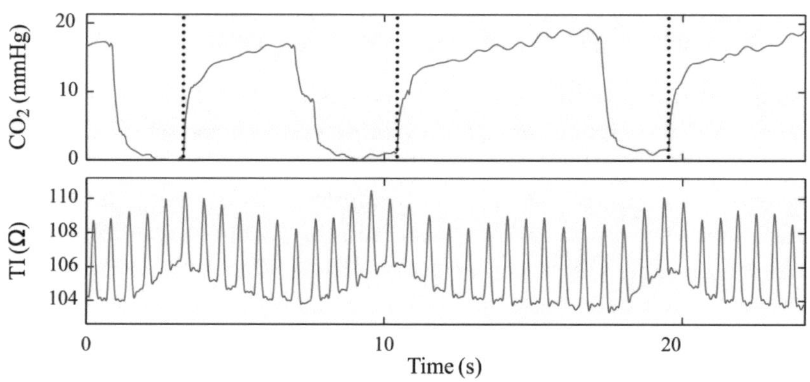

Figure 5. A segment of an episode of the dataset. From top to bottom, the capnogram and the TI. The black dotted lines represent the ventilations annotated in the capnogram.

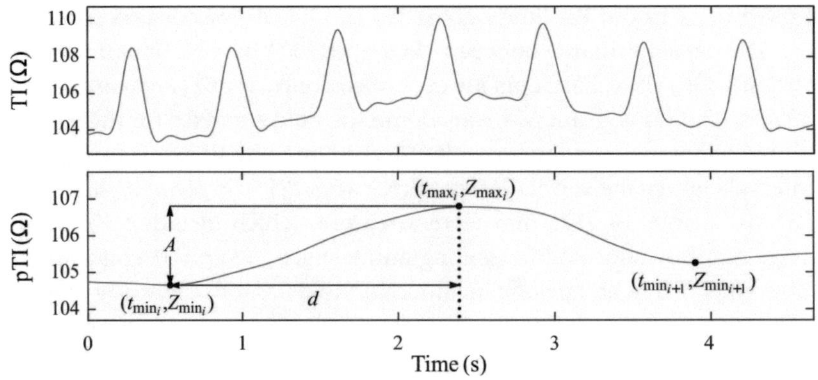

Figure 6. A short segment showing how preprocessing reveals the fluctuation caused by a ventilation. The inflation amplitude, *A*, and inflation time, *d*, are depicted as well as the local maximum and minima.

were also computed, namely the mean ventilation rate and the FMH, the latter to evaluate hyperventilation.

2.2. Evaluation of the ventilation detector

The feasibility and accuracy of the TI signal as a surrogate of the capnogram to measure ventilation metrics was evaluated using the test set. Distributions for each metric obtained from the TI and from the capnogram were analyzed independently applying the one sample Kolmogorov-Smirnov normality test. For normal distributions, the two-sample t-test was performed to test for equal means, and for not normal distributions, the Mann-Whitney U test was used to test for equal medians. The limits of agreement (LOA) between the values obtained from the TI and from the capnogram were analyzed using Bland-Altman plots for each metric.

The ventilation detector showed a median (interquartile range) SE of 92.2% (87.4–95.8), and a median PPV of 81.0% (67.2–90.5). These scores are similar to those reported by other authors as Risdal et al. [35] and Edelson et al. [34]. Nevertheless the proposed method was tested with an independent gold standard, annotated in the capnogram, and it requires a much simpler processing which would permit an easier integration in an AED.

Table 1 is a summary of the ventilation quality metrics computed from the TI and compared to those obtained from the capnogram. Data are presented as mean (standard deviation). The distributions of the FMH obtained from the TI and capnogram were not normal, although they did have equal medians ($p = 0.66$). Mean and instantaneous ventilation rates came from normal distributions. The mean ventilation rate and the FMH obtained from TI and capnogram showed equal means, with mean errors of 1.54 min^{-1} and 1%. That was not the case for the instantaneous ventilation rate, with different mean ($p < 0.001$) and a mean error of 3.30 min^{-1}.

Figure 7 shows the Bland-Altman plots for each ventilation quality metric, and the corresponding 95% LOA depicted with horizontal lines. For the quality metrics, both the mean

Metric	Gold standard	TI	Error	p
Mean ventilation rate (min^{-1})	9.54 (2.94)	10.87 (2.68)	1.54 (1.44)	0.07
FMH (%)	11.39 (18.35)	10.09(16.88)	1.29 (2.59)	0.66*
Instantaneous ventilation rate (min^{-1})	10.23 (4.29)	13.09 (4.52)	3.30 (2.88)	<0.001

*The p-values obtained from the t-test and Mann–Whitney U test are expressed for each metric.

Table 1. Mean (SD) values computed from the gold standard and from the TI for each ventilation quality metric and the error.

ventilation rate and the FMH showed minor errors, with small LOAs. These results support the use of the TI to accurately evaluate the ventilation metrics when debriefing resuscitation episodes.

The Bland Altman plot for the instantaneous ventilation rate showed large LOAs, in the range of −8 to 5 ventilations per minute. These results question the accuracy of the method based on the TI to monitor the ventilation rate every 15 s.

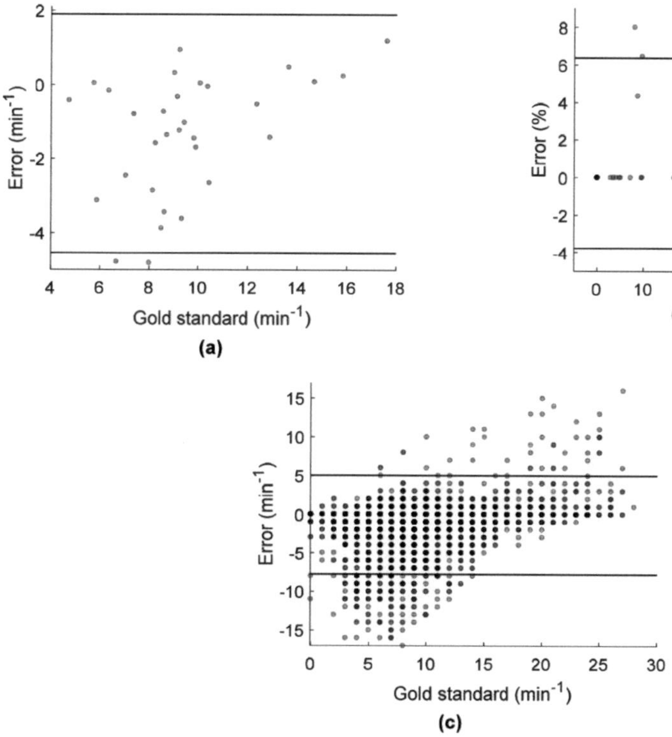

Figure 7. Bland-Altman plots for mean ventilation rate, FMH, and instantaneous ventilation rate are represented in a, b, and c panels respectively. The 95% LOA is depicted in black dashed lines.

3. The use of capnography to monitor ventilation rate

Capnography is a noninvasive monitoring technique that shows the partial pressure of the exhaled CO_2 of the patient over the time [36]. The initial use of the capnography signal (or capnogram) was for anesthesia monitoring, but its use has expanded to other fields such as emergency medicine as it provides information about CO_2 production levels, lung perfusion and alveolar ventilation among others [37]. Current resuscitation guidelines recommend the use of capnography to confirm endotracheal intubation, detect return of spontaneous circulation, monitor the effectiveness of chest compressions and monitor ventilation rate [8].

Advanced monitor/defibrillators used by medical personnel include modules that show the capnogram of the patient during CPR. In current commercial equipment, two main acquisition techniques are used: mainstream and sidestream capnography [38]. The mainstream technology has an infrared light sensor which is placed directly in the main way of expired flow to measure the absorption of CO_2. In sidestream, the expired gases are continuously aspirated from a 1–2 m long sampling tube, and the sensor is placed at the end. **Figure 8** shows the general structure of both acquisition technologies.

The capnogram shows the evolution of the CO_2 expired during the ventilations provided to the patient in cardiac arrest, where the cycle of every ventilation is visible. Four phases are visible in the cycle of each ventilation [39], as illustrated in **Figure 9**: the inspiration baseline (phase I), the expiration upstroke (phase II), the expiratory plateau (phase III) and the expiration down stroke (phase IV). The maximum value observed in the third phase is the so-called $EtCO_2$ (End-tidal CO_2). In hemodynamically stable patients, the value is about 35–45 mmHg, similar to the partial pressure of the CO_2 in the blood [37, 41]. During cardiac arrest, the elimination of CO_2 is reduced and it is accumulated in the tissues. This is because an abrupt

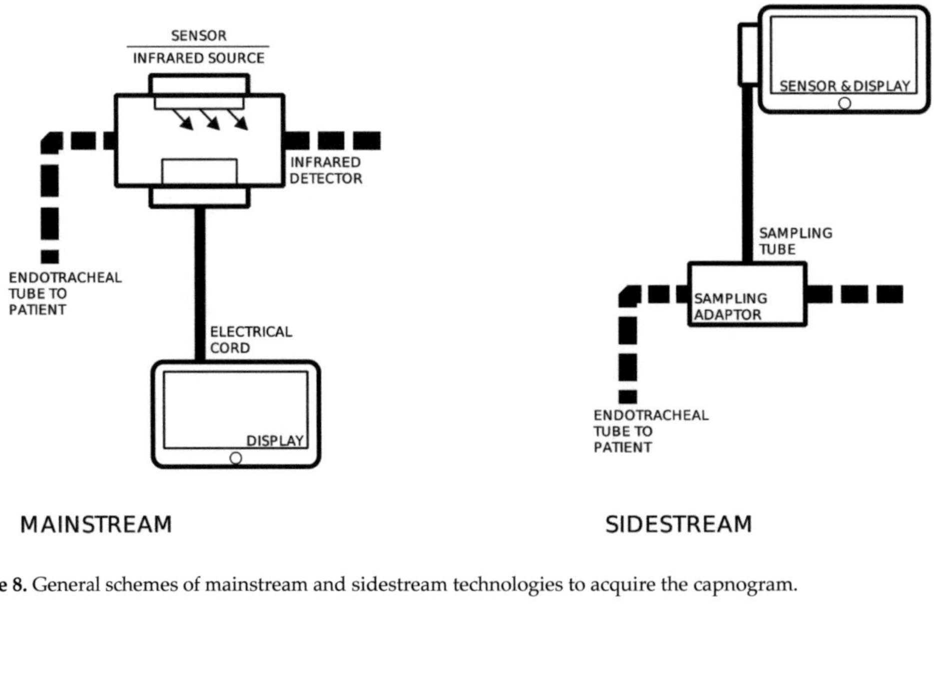

Figure 8. General schemes of mainstream and sidestream technologies to acquire the capnogram.

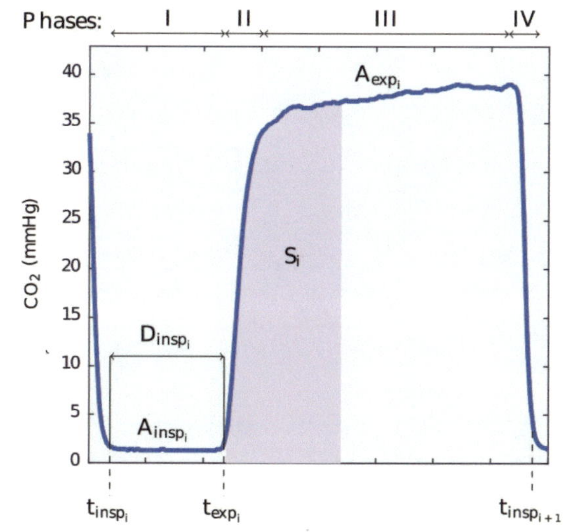

Figure 9. Basic waveform of the capnography signal during a cycle of ventilation. Four phases of the cycle and the features for automatic ventilation detection are shown. Adapted from [40].

decrease in cardiac output implies a reduced CO_2 transportation from the tissues to the lungs, and therefore $EtCO_2$ values decrease almost to zero. Effective chest compressions or recovering pulse make this value increase [42, 43].

During CPR, chest compressions may induce artifacts that corrupt the capnogram. Idris et al. [44] analyzed 210 patients and they detected artifacts in the capnography signal in 154 of 210 episodes, an incidence of 73.3%. More recently, Leturiondo et al. [45] reported an incidence of 42% (99 of 232 episodes showed artifacts). The source and level of the corruption is not well defined yet, and depends on both the patient and the way CPR is performed. Bottom panels of the cases represented in **Figure 10** show examples of the capnogram for four patients, uncorrupted in panels a and c, and corrupted by chest compression artifact in panels b and d. The interference caused by chest compressions complicate the design of automatic ventilation detection algorithms based on the capnogram that would permit the monitoring of ventilation rate and the retrospective debriefing of resuscitation episodes.

The first algorithm to automatically detect ventilations during CPR in the capnogram was proposed by Edelson et al. [34]. They used both the capnogram and the impedance signal to detect the ventilation instants, combining two finite-state-machines. The capnogram-based algorithm provided SE/PPV of 82%/91%. A similar algorithm was proposed by Leturiondo et al. [45] based exclusively on the capnogram with SE/PPV above 95% for uncorrupted intervals, and the accuracy decreased during chest compressions. Both proposals [34, 45] developed the algorithm using as ground truth the ventilations annotated manually in the impedance signal. As it can be observed in **Figure 10** the impedance signal is highly affected by the CPR artifact, and the amplitude of the fluctuations caused by ventilations is not constant, it has been reported to be nonlinear with the tidal volume for all the population [31]. Both factors question the reliability of the ground truth used to evaluate the algorithms.

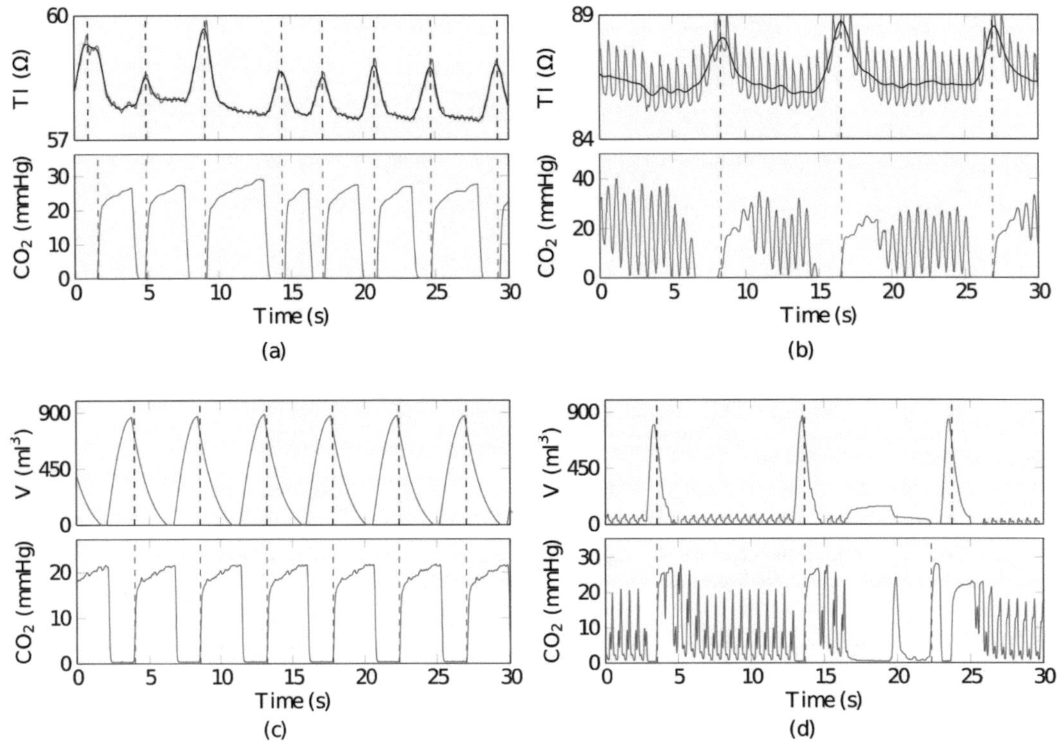

Figure 10. Examples of the capnogram (bottom) and the signal used to annotate the gold standard ventilations (top) are shown for the OHD (panels a and b) and for the IHD (panels c and d). For the OHD, the raw impedance signal (blue) and the filtered impedance signal (black) are shown, and for the IHD the volume signal. In both cases, black vertical lines show the annotated ventilations in the gold standard, and red vertical lines the detected ventilations in the capnogram.

3.1. An automated ventilation detector based on the capnogram

This section describes an algorithm developed using the gas exchange flow measured by a ventilator to annotate the ground truth for the ventilations instants [40]. To the best of our knowledge, this is the only ventilation detector tested with the most reliable ground truth.

Two datasets were used to develop and test the algorithm: an In-Hospital Dataset (IHD) and Out-of-Hospital Dataset (OHD). A total of 83 episodes (62 in-hospital and 21 out-of-hospital) were considered with a duration of 4880 min. The episodes included 16,899 and 29,841 ventilations, with a percentage of 38 and 8% of the time with compressions for the OHD and the IHD, respectively. The general characteristics of both datasets are summarized in **Table 2**. Each episode of the IHD contained the capnogram, and the airflow and air volume signals provided by the ventilator; the instants of the ventilations were annotated based on the volume of the flow signal, as shown in **Figure 10**. Chest compression intervals were identified by medical annotations and abrupt increases in arterial blood pressure. The cases in the OHD included the capnogram, the TI and the CD signals. The CD was used to identify chest compression intervals, while TI and CD were the ground truth to mark ventilations manually. **Figure 10** shows epochs of episodes included in both datasets. For each panel, the top figure shows the independent gold standard (volume signal for IHD and the thoracic impedance signal for OHD), and in the bottom the capnography. The ventilations

Parameter	OHD	IHD
Number of episodes	62	21
Total duration (min)	2545	2335
Total number of ventilations (% with CPR)	16,899 (38)	29,841 (8)
Instantaneous ventilation rate (min^{-1})	9.9 (8.7–13.1)	14.3 (12.6–18.2)
Minutes with hyperventilation per episode (%)	10 (2–35)	14 (0–88)

The instantaneous ventilation rate and minutes with hyperventilation are given per episode as median (interquartile range).

Table 2. Characteristics of both out-of-hospital (OHD) and in-hospital (IHD) datasets.

marked in the gold standard are depicted with black dashed lines. Both gold standards show fluctuations concurrently with the capnography signal for each ventilation. A total of 37 episodes randomly selected from the OHD dataset were used to design and train the algorithm; the test set was conformed with the remaining 25 cases of the OHD and the 21 IHD cases.

The method relies on the computation of the values corresponding to the features shown in **Figure 9**. First, the signal is preprocessed with a low-pass filter with a cutoff frequency of 10 Hz; then values of the waveform below 5 mmHg are set to zero. Potential ventilations are detected between the start of inspiration, t_{insp} (insufflation during ventilation), and the start of expiration, t_{exp} (deflation during ventilation). Both instants are computed based on the positive and negative peaks in the first difference of the signal. Then the following six features, depicted in **Figure 9** are computed:

- Duration of inspiration baseline, D_{insp}.
- Mean value of the signal during plateau, A_{exp}.
- Area of the first second of the expiratory plateau, S_{exp}.
- Relative increase of the signal, computed as:

$$A_r = \frac{A_{\exp} - A_{insp}}{A_{\exp}}, \tag{1}$$

where A_{insp} is the mean amplitude of the signal during inspiration baseline.

- Interval between actual potential ventilation and the last detected ventilation, t_{ref}.

The algorithm discriminates real ventilations based on fixed thresholds for D_{insp} and t_{ref}, and adaptive thresholds for A_{exp}, S_{exp} and A_r. The adaptation for the kth ventilation was computed based on the last p ventilations according to the following equation:

$$Th_k = \frac{w}{p} \sum_{n=k-p}^{k} x_n, \tag{2}$$

where w is a weighting factor between 0 and 1 and x_n represents the value of the feature for ventilation n. A more detailed description of the algorithm can be found in [40]. **Figure 10** shows examples of the algorithm performance. The black dashed lines represent the manual ventilation annotations in the gold standard, and the red dashed lines correspond to the ventilations detected by the algorithm.

As for the TI-based detector, the detected ventilations were used to compute the instantaneous ventilation rate, and the global ventilation metrics per episode.

3.2. Evaluation of the ventilation detector

The algorithm showed overall SE and PPV values above 99% and 97%, respectively. For the OHD, the median (interquartile range) SE and PPV per patient were 99.1 (96.9–99.8)% and 97.0 (95.9–98.9)%. When only the intervals with chest compressions were considered the SE and PPV were 99.0 (95.7–100)% and 97.6(94.8–100)%. For the IHD, SE and PPV were 100 (99.8–100)% and 100 (99.8–100)%. During compressions the performance dropped slightly to 99.8 (98.7–100)% and 98.3 (92.9–100)%, respectively.

The concordance correlation coefficient on ventilation rate measured as proposed in [46] was higher than 0.98 for both datasets, even during chest compressions. **Figure 11** shows the

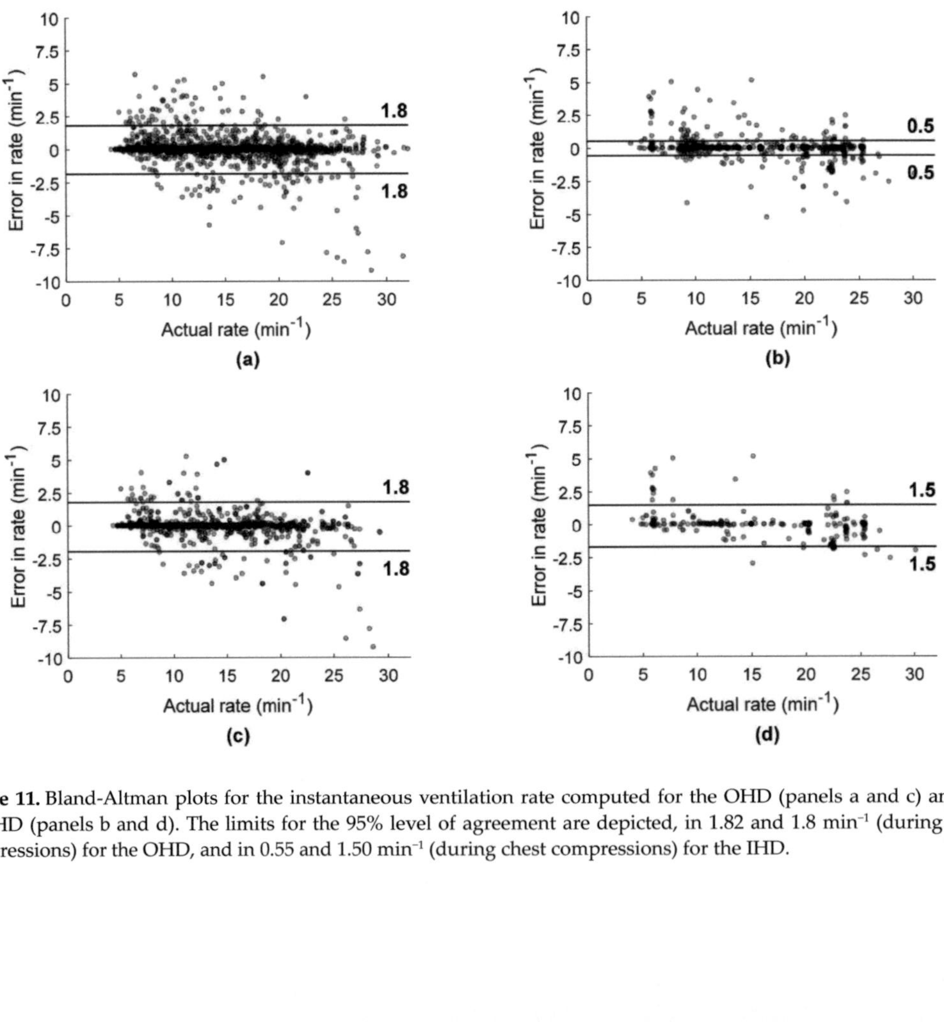

Figure 11. Bland-Altman plots for the instantaneous ventilation rate computed for the OHD (panels a and c) and for the IHD (panels b and d). The limits for the 95% level of agreement are depicted, in 1.82 and 1.8 min^{-1} (during chest compressions) for the OHD, and in 0.55 and 1.50 min^{-1} (during chest compressions) for the IHD.

	Gold standard	Algorithm	p
OHD			
Mean ventilation rate (min^{-1})	11.74 (10.34–15.47)	12.11 (10.56–15.37)	0.88
FMH (%)	2.56 (0–34.77)	2.50 (0–34.51)	0.94
Instantaneous ventilation rate (min^{-1})	9.07 (12.44–17.28)	9.23 (12.56–17.31)	0.79
IHD			
Mean ventilation rate (min^{-1})	14.02 (12.53–17.70)	14.02 (12.48–17.77)	1
FMH (%)	5.49 (0–81.08)	5.48 (0–80.39)	1
Instantaneous ventilation rate (min^{-1})	13.98 (12.98–18.98)	13.98 (12.98–18.98)	0.52

All p values were calculated using Mann-Whitney U test.

Table 3. Median (interquartile range) values computed from the gold standard and from the capnogram for each ventilation quality metric.

Bland-Altman plots and the 95% LOA between the gold standard and the algorithm, which was lower than 1.85 in any case. These results show that this capnogram-based method reliably estimates the instantaneous rate.

The detailed results for the ventilation quality metrics are shown in **Table 3**. It can be observed that the mean ventilation rate and the FMH showed equal distributions ($p > 0.05$) when compared to the ground truth for both the OHD and IHD episodes. The unsigned errors were close to zero for both metrics and for both datasets. These results support the use of this method to retrospectively debrief resuscitation episodes.

4. Discussion and conclusions

In this chapter, the monitoring of ventilations provided during out-of-hospital CPR was addressed with two objectives. First, giving feedback on the instantaneous ventilation rate to rescuers. Second, to allow retrospectively evaluation of ventilation rates and hyperventilation metrics during resuscitation episodes.

The analysis focused on the feasibility of the TI acquired by the defibrillation pads, and the capnogram to accurately report feedback on ventilation. Methods based exclusively on each of the signals were proposed and statistically evaluated. These methods could be integrated in commercial defibrillation equipment, the TI-based algorithm in any AED or monitor/defibrillators, and the capnogram-based algorithm in any equipment that includes capnography.

Several aspects deserved attention in the development of the algorithms. In the setting of the procedure, the gold standard was carefully selected. In the case of the TI, manual annotations were defined in the capnogram, as a result of the consensus of three experts. In the case of the capnogram, the independent signal used as gold standard was the gas volume exchanged measured by an external ventilator. In both cases, the gold standard was annotated using an independent signal, including the gas exchange information, which is, in our opinion, the most reliable signal. This is a key factor when evaluating the accuracy and reliability of the methods.

In any case, the simplicity of the method was a priority. The algorithms proposed do not rely on complicated or computationally intensive signal processing techniques, so they could be integrated in current defibrillation equipment without much increase of computational requirements.

The scores obtained for the TI-based method are similar to those previously reported in terms of SE (around 90%), and slightly below for PPV. For the capnogram-based method, SE/PPV was both above 97% in any dataset, even when chest compressions were provided.

Both methods are valid to be integrated in the software provided to retrospectively review the quality of the ventilations. Errors below 2 min^{-1} in the mean rate and about 1% in the FMH for both the TI and the capnogram are sufficient for an accurate retrospective evaluation. The integration of these methods in the revision software provided by commercial equipment would permit debriefing on ventilation after cardiac arrest. The American Heart Association emphasizes the post-even analysis of the data, which contributes to the continuous quality improvement, closing the gap between the ideal and the actual performance of OHCA resuscitation. Excessive ventilation rates are often observed during CPR both out- and in-hospital cardiac arrest [14], and code team debriefing with audiovisual feedback has been associated with a decrease in mean ventilation rates from 18 to 13 min^{-1} [34, 47].

For the audiovisual feedback to the rescuer, the instantaneous rate should be provided to the rescuers, associated, if necessary with hyperventilation alarms. The instantaneous rate, as computed in the methods proposed, would permit feedback every 15 s, which is a reasonable compromise to follow the feedback and adhere to the recommendations of the guidelines. The method proposed on the capnogram was very reliable with errors below 2 min^{-1} for any dataset even during chest compressions. That was not the case for the TI, as the mean error for the instantaneous rate was above 3 min^{-1}. Two are the reasons that make difficult the automated detection of ventilations in the TI. First, the fluctuations caused by ventilations are very variable, even for the same patient, so adaptive thresholding is required for the algorithm. Panel a in **Figure 10** shows clear examples in which similar ventilation cycles in the capnogram appear with very different amplitudes in the impedance waveform. Therefore, it is very difficult to define a universally valid TI amplitude threshold for the detection of ventilations. Second, artifacts caused by chest compressions and other noise make difficult to automatically detect every ventilation.

Finally, it should be stated that the results and conclusions presented in this chapter are limited by the specific characteristics of the data used. Using the TI or the capnogram from other equipment, with different electronic circuitry and defibrillation pads, may require readapting the values and thresholds of the algorithms and may result in different values of the performance metrics.

Acknowledgements

This work has been partially supported by the Spanish Ministerio de Economía y Competividad, jointly with the Fondo Europeo de Desarrollo Regional (FEDER), project TEC2015-64678-R, by the University of the Basque Country via project EHU16/18, the Ayudas a Grupos de Investigación GIU17/031 and the unit UFI11/16, and by the Basque Government through the grant PRE_2017_1_0112.

Author details

Andoni Elola, Erik Alonso, Elisabete Aramendi* and Unai Irusta

*Address all correspondence to: elisabete.aramendi@ehu.es

University of the Basque Country, Bilbao, Spain

References

[1] Zheng Z-J, Croft JB, Giles WH, Mensah GA. Sudden cardiac death in the United States, 1989 to 1998. Circulation. 2001;**104**(18):2158-2163

[2] Atwood C, Eisenberg MS, Herlitz J, Rea TD. Incidence of EMS-treated out-of-hospital cardiac arrest in Europe. Resuscitation. 2005;**67**(1):75-80

[3] Bayés de Luna A, Coumel P, Leclercq JF. Ambulatory sudden cardiac death: Mechanisms of production of fatal arrhythmia on the basis of data from 157 cases. American Heart Journal. 1989;**117**(1):151-159

[4] Cobb LA, Fahrenbruch CE, Olsufka M, Copass MK. Changing incidence of out-of-hospital ventricular fibrillation, 1980-2000. Journal of the American Medical Association. 2002;**288**(23):3008-3013

[5] Chugh SS, Jui J, Gunson K, Stecker EC, John BT, Thompson B, et al. Current burden of sudden cardiac death: Multiple source surveillance versus retrospective death certificate-based review in a large U.S. community. Journal of the American College of Cardiology. 2004;**44**(6):1268-1275

[6] Rea TD, Eisenberg MS, Sinibaldi G, White RD. Incidence of EMS-treated out-of-hospital cardiac arrest in the United States. Resuscitation. 2004;**63**(1):17-24

[7] Larsen MP, Eisenberg MS, Cummins RO, Hallstrom AP. Predicting survival from out-of-hospital cardiac arrest: A graphic model. Annals of Emergency Medicine. 1993;**22**(11):1652-1658

[8] Soar J, Nolan JP, Böttiger BW, Perkins GD, Lott C, Carli P, et al. European resuscitation council guidelines for resuscitation 2015: Section 3. Adult advanced life support. Resuscitation. 2015;**95**:100-147

[9] Koster RW, Baubin MA, Bossaert LL, Caballero A, Cassan P, Castrén M, et al. European resuscitation council guidelines for resuscitation 2010 section 2. Adult basic life support and use of automated external defibrillators. Resuscitation. 2010;**81**(10):1277-1292

[10] Bag-Mask Ventilation Fails to Improve on Endotracheal Intubation in Cardiac Arre [Internet]. [cited 2018 Jan 29]. Available from: https://www.escardio.org/The-ESC/Press-Office/Press-releases/bag-mask-ventilation-fails-to-improve-on-endotracheal-intubation-in-cardiac-arrest

[11] Berg RA, Hemphill R, Abella BS, Aufderheide TP, Cave DM, Hazinski MF, et al. Part 5: Adult basic life support: 2010 American Heart Association Guidelines for Cardiopulmonary Resuscitation and Emergency Cardiovascular Care. Circulation. 2010;**122**(18 Suppl 3):S685-S705

[12] Abella BS, Alvarado JP, Myklebust H, Edelson DP, Barry A, O'Hearn N, et al. Quality of cardiopulmonary resuscitation during in-hospital cardiac arrest. Journal of the American Medical Association. 2005;**293**(3):305-310

[13] McInnes AD, Sutton RM, Orioles A, Nishisaki A, Niles D, Abella BS, et al. The first quantitative report of ventilation rate during in-hospital resuscitation of older children and adolescents. Resuscitation. 2011;**82**(8):1025-1029

[14] Aufderheide TP, Sigurdsson G, Pirrallo RG, Yannopoulos D, McKnite S, von Briesen C, et al. Hyperventilation-induced hypotension during cardiopulmonary resuscitation. Circulation. 2004;**109**(16):1960-1965

[15] O'Neill JF, Deakin CD. Do we hyperventilate cardiac arrest patients? Resuscitation. 2007;**73**(1):82-85

[16] Milander MM, Hiscok PS, Sanders AB, Kern KB, Berg RA, Ewy GA. Chest compression and ventilation rates during cardiopulmonary resuscitation: The effects of audible tone guidance. Academic Emergency Medicine: Official Journal of the Society for Academic Emergency Medicine. 1995;**2**(8):708-713

[17] Woodson RD. Physiological significance of oxygen dissociation curve shifts. Critical Care Medicine. 1979;**7**(9):368-373

[18] Madden JA. The effect of carbon dioxide on cerebral arteries. Pharmacology & Therapeutics. 1993;**59**(2):229-250

[19] Karlsson T, Stjernström EL, Stjernström H, Norlén K, Wiklund L. Central and regional blood flow during hyperventilation. An experimental study in the pig. Acta Anaesthesiologica Scandinavica. 1994;**38**(2):180-186

[20] Yannopoulos D, McKnite S, Aufderheide TP, Sigurdsson G, Pirrallo RG, Benditt D, et al. Effects of incomplete chest wall decompression during cardiopulmonary resuscitation on coronary and cerebral perfusion pressures in a porcine model of cardiac arrest. Resuscitation. 2005;**64**(3):363-372

[21] Kramer-Johansen J, Edelson DP, Losert H, Köhler K, Abella BS. Uniform reporting of measured quality of cardiopulmonary resuscitation (CPR). Resuscitation. 2007;**74**(3):406-417

[22] Kerber RE, Grayzel J, Hoyt R, Marcus M, Kennedy J. Transthoracic resistance in human defibrillation. Influence of body weight, chest size, serial shocks, paddle size and paddle contact pressure. Circulation. 1981;**63**(3):676-682

[23] Gruben KG. Mechanics of pressure generation during cardiopulmonary resuscitation [thesis]. 1994

[24] Fitzgibbon E, Berger R, Tsitlik J, Halperin HR. Determination of the noise source in the electrocardiogram during cardiopulmonary resuscitation. Critical Care Medicine. 2002;**30**(4):S148-S153

[25] Stecher FS, Olsen J-A, Stickney RE, Wik L. Transthoracic impedance used to evaluate performance of cardiopulmonary resuscitation during out of hospital cardiac arrest. Resuscitation. 2008;**79**(3):432-437

[26] Losert H, Risdal M, Sterz F, Nysaether J, Köhler K, Eftestøl T, et al. Thoracic impedance changes measured via defibrillator pads can monitor ventilation in critically ill patients and during cardiopulmonary resuscitation. Critical Care Medicine. 2006;**34**(9):2399-2405

[27] Pellis T, Bisera J, Tang W, Weil MH. Expanding automatic external defibrillators to include automated detection of cardiac, respiratory, and cardiorespiratory arrest. Critical Care Medicine. 2002;**30**(4):S176-S178

[28] Alonso E, Aramendi E, Daya M, Irusta U, Chicote B, Russell JK, et al. Circulation detection using the electrocardiogram and the thoracic impedance acquired by defibrillation pads. Resuscitation. 2016;**99**:56-62

[29] Alonso E, Ruiz J, Aramendi E, González-Otero D, de Gauna SR, Ayala U, et al. Reliability and accuracy of the thoracic impedance signal for measuring cardiopulmonary resuscitation quality metrics. Resuscitation. 2015;**88**:28-34

[30] Hull E, Irie T, Heemstra H, Wildevuur CR. Transthoracic electrical impedance: Artifacts associated with electrode movement. Resuscitation. 1978;**6**(2):115-124

[31] Roberts K, Srinivasan V, Niles DE, Eilevstjønn J, Tyler L, Boyle L, et al. Does change in thoracic impedance measured via defibrillator electrode pads accurately detect ventilation breaths in children? Resuscitation. 2010;**81**(11):1544-1549

[32] Risdal M, Aase SO, Kramer-Johansen J, Eftesøl T. Automatic identification of return of spontaneous circulation during cardiopulmonary resuscitation. IEEE Transactions on Biomedical Engineering. 2008;**55**(1):60-68

[33] Husoy J, Eilevstjønn J, Eftestøl T, Aase SO, Myklebust H, Steen PA. Removal of cardiopulmonary resuscitation artifacts from human ECG using an efficient matching pursuit-like algorithm. IEEE Transactions on Biomedical Engineering. 2002;**49**(11):1287-1298

[34] Edelson DP, Eilevstjønn J, Weidman EK, Retzer E, Hoek TLV, Abella BS. Capnography and chest-wall impedance algorithms for ventilation detection during cardiopulmonary resuscitation. Resuscitation. 2010;**81**(3):317-322

[35] Risdal M, Aase SO, Stavland M, Eftestøl T. Impedance-based ventilation detection during cardiopulmonary resuscitation. IEEE Transactions on Biomedical Engineering. 2007;**54**(12):2237-2245

[36] Terndrup TE, Rhee J. Available ventilation monitoring methods during pre-hospital cardiopulmonary resuscitation. Resuscitation. 2006;**71**(1):10-18

[37] Sanders AB. Capnometry in emergency medicine. Annals of Emergency Medicine. 1989;**18**(12):1287-1290

[38] Jaffe MB. Mainstream or sidestream capnography? Environment. 2002;**4**:5

[39] Pantazopoulos C, Xanthos T, Pantazopoulos I, Papalois A, Kouskouni E, Iacovidou N. A review of carbon dioxide monitoring during adult cardiopulmonary resuscitation. Heart, Lung & Circulation. 2015;**24**(11):1053-1061

[40] Aramendi E, Elola A, Alonso E, Irusta U, Daya M, Russell JK, et al. Feasibility of the capnogram to monitor ventilation rate during cardiopulmonary resuscitation. Resuscitation. 2017;**110**:162-168

[41] Trilĺo G, von Planta M, Kette F. ETCO2 monitoring during low flow states: Clinical aims and limits. Resuscitation. 1994;**27**(1):1-8

[42] Sheak KR, Wiebe DJ, Leary M, Babaeizadeh S, Yuen TC, Zive D, et al. Quantitative relationship between end-tidal carbon dioxide and CPR quality during both in-hospital and out-of-hospital cardiac arrest. Resuscitation. 2015;**89**:149-154

[43] Pokorná M, Nečas E, Kratochvíl J, Skřipský R, Andrlík M, Franěk O. A sudden increase in partial pressure end-tidal carbon dioxide (PETCO2) at the moment of return of spontaneous circulation. The Journal of Emergency Medicine. 2010;**38**(5):614-621

[44] Idris AH, Daya M, Owens P, O'Neill S, Helfenbein ED, Babaeizadeh S, et al. Abstract 83: High incidence of chest compression oscillations associated with capnography during out-of-hospital cardiopulmonary resuscitation. Circulation. 2010;**122**(21 Supplement):A83

[45] Leturiondo M, de Gauna SR, Ruiz JM, Gutiérrez JJ, Leturiondo LA, González-Otero DM, et al. Influence of chest compression artefact on capnogram-based ventilation detection during out-of-hospital cardiopulmonary resuscitation. Resuscitation. 2018;**124**:63-68

[46] Lin LI. A concordance correlation coefficient to evaluate reproducibility. Biometrics. 1989;**45**(1):255-268

[47] Morrison LJ, Neumar RW, Zimmerman JL, Link MS, Newby LK, McMullan PW, et al. Strategies for improving survival after in-hospital cardiac arrest in the United States: 2013 consensus recommendations: A consensus statement from the American Heart Association. Circulation. 2013;**127**(14):1538-1563

Chapter 5

Non-Invasive Ventilation of the Neonate

Omid Fathi, Amy Brown Schlegel and
Edward G. Shepherd

Additional information is available at the end of the chapter

http://dx.doi.org/10.5772/intechopen.72395

Abstract

The use of mechanical ventilation in the past few decades has greatly contributed to the survival of critically ill neonates, both preterm and term. With this, however, has come an accompanied rise in certain complications and neonatal co-morbidities. Avoiding mechanical ventilation, or at least minimizing the time a neonate is intubated, is considered a critical goal in the care of these patients. Different modes of non-invasive ventilation have developed over the course of the time to help address these issues.

Keywords: non-invasive ventilation, neonate, preterm, prematurity, continuous positive airway pressure (CPAP), bilevel positive airway pressure (BiPAP), nasal intermittent positive pressure ventilation (NIPPV), high flow nasal cannula (HFNC)

1. Introduction

Survival of premature infants has improved steadily since neonatal care became a national focus in the 1960's. A key component in this improvement is improved respiratory care, especially mechanical ventilation. Increased survival of vulnerable infants, however, is associated with complications and co-morbidities, some of which are directly caused by invasive ventilation. Therefore, minimizing exposure to mechanical ventilation is critical to the care of these babies. Gregory et al., in 1971, first described the use of continuous positive airway pressure (CPAP) to treat neonates afflicted with respiratory distress syndrome (RDS), which transformed respiratory care of neonates [1]. Subsequently, the use of CPAP and other forms of non-invasive ventilation have become the standard of care and have saved countless lives.

Non-invasive ventilation refers to any mode of respiratory support provided via the nasal airway of infants to support spontaneous breathing, without placement of an endotracheal tube. The most common non-invasive modes include nasal continuous positive airway pressure (NCPAP), non-invasive intermittent mandatory ventilation (NIMV), and humidified high-flow nasal cannula (HHFNC). The ultimate goal of each of these devices is to prevent barotrauma, volutrauma, and atelectotrauma, all of which contribute to lung injury and long-term complications. Proposed mechanisms of lung protection due to non-invasive ventilation include mitigation of shear-type injury by maintenance of optimal end-expiratory lung volumes and prevention of cyclical collapse and over-distention of alveoli. Other potential benefits include lung-recruitment, improved gas exchange, and decreased work of breathing [2].

In this chapter, we will first explore historical aspects of the development of non-invasive ventilation in neonates. Then we will focus on specific respiratory mechanics unique to neonates and post-uterine adaptation. Finally, we will discuss specific non-invasive modalities.

2. Historical perspectives

Improved perinatal care, the advent of parenteral nutrition, advances in thermoregulation, and aggressive neonatal resuscitation have all contributed enormously to improved outcomes for neonates. Perhaps the most significant change, however, is a marked improvement in our ability to provide aggressive and sophisticated respiratory care and support to ever-smaller infants. In this section, we will focus on the historical development of innovative approaches to non-invasive ventilation in tiny premature infants.

Although Gregory et al. published the first modern description of the use of CPAP to treat RDS, a similar device was first described in 1914 by Professor August Ritter von Reuss [2]. This device resembled bubble CPAP, and consisted of an oxygen tank with tubing attached to the equivalent of a mask-and-bag device, with a simple valve to regulate oxygen flow. Unfortunately, it took almost six decades for this concept to gain acceptance. Prior to Gregory's description of CPAP, there was very little respiratory support that could be provided to neonates. In the 1940s and 1950s, the provision of supplemental oxygen was the sole therapeutic option for ill neonates [3]. It was during this time that two seminal discoveries were made. The first was the discovery that supplemental oxygen provided benefit to ill neonates, but that exposure to high concentrations led to blindness due to retinopathy of prematurity (ROP) [3]. The second was a report by Avery and Mead in 1959 describing increased surface tension in lung fluid recovered from preterm babies that had died from respiratory distress syndrome, and the observation that preterm infants lacked some sort of "surface-active agent" that could alleviate these forces [4].

Neonatology was still a relatively new field in the latter part of the 20th century, and 1963 was a pivotal year in its development. President John F. Kennedy's son, Patrick Bouvier Kennedy, was born 6 weeks prematurely and died from complications of respiratory distress syndrome on the third day of life [3]. This inspired rapid innovation in the development of new technologies geared towards critically ill neonates. Infant ventilators, blood gas machines, umbilical vascular catheterization and the development of the first true neonatal intensive care units all occurred in the late 1960s. As the field improved, survival rates for neonates with respiratory compromise began to improve as well, mainly due to the widespread use of infant ventilators.

Unfortunately, these advances were also associated with complications and many of these neonates were left with a form of chronic lung disease. This was first described in 1967 by Northway et al., who noted that prolonged exposure to mechanical ventilation and supplemental oxygen were likely to blame [5].

Subsequently, in 1971, Gregory et al., described the use of CPAP to treat neonates with respiratory distress syndrome, using either an endotracheal tube or a head box [2]. This use of CPAP represented an intermediate step that was more supportive than supplemental oxygen alone, was relatively easy to use, and seemed to avoid exposure to the injury associated with mechanical ventilation. The introduction of CPAP in neonates was not the only milestone that this decade produced; in 1972, Liggins and Howie published the results of a randomized controlled trial of antenatal steroids in mothers expected to delivery premature infants. They demonstrated that steroids accelerated fetal lung maturation and decreased the risk of respiratory distress syndrome and death by as much as half [3].

Despite the successes associated with CPAP and antenatal steroids, there were substantial concerns about risks. Specifically, some observers suggested that air leaks and pneumothoraces were more common with CPAP than mechanical ventilation. In addition, CPAP seemed to lead to gastric and abdominal distention of unclear clinical significance. Finally, there were fears that the devices themselves would predispose infants to neurological and cosmetic injury [2]. For these among other reasons, intermittent mandatory ventilation using an endotracheal tube was widely adopted, and quickly overtook CPAP as the standard of respiratory care for critically ill neonates. In addition, for about two decades, CPAP was largely replaced by non-invasive intermittent mandatory ventilation (NIMV). It involved using time-cycled, pressure-controlled breaths delivered by a mechanical ventilator via an oronasal mask or prongs [2].

In the late 1980s, there was renewed interest in CPAP and non-invasive ventilation, sparked by the seminal report in 1987 by Avery et al. which concluded that, among eight NICUs observed, the center with the most aggressive use of NCPAP had the lowest rates of chronic lung disease [6]. Coupled with the fact that the landscape of chronic lung disease, as originally described in 1967, was changing in both a clinical and histological sense due to prolonged exposure to mechanical ventilation, it was no surprise that non-invasive ventilation was resurgent. While CPAP was originally designed for the premature baby with respiratory distress syndrome, today it has multiple uses in neonates of varying ages and conditions. It is used to successfully treat transient tachypnea of the newborn, congenital pneumonia, meconium aspiration syndrome, primary pulmonary hypertension, as well as central apnea of prematurity and certain congenital upper airway lesions [2]. While the technology has certainly evolved quite a bit since Professor von Reuss' initial apparatus in 1914, CPAP and other forms of non-invasive ventilation have become the cornerstones of neonatal respiratory care.

3. Neonatal pulmonary mechanics

It is important to understand the core concepts of fetal and neonatal lung development, as well as basic pulmonary mechanics, to better understand the most appropriate respiratory support modality. Fundamentally, the respiratory system is designed for the conduction and humidification of air into the lungs, uptake of oxygen from the ambient environment, and the removal of waste product in the form of carbon dioxide. All of this ensures that normal aerobic cellular metabolism is supported and that acid–base homeostasis is maintained.

The respiratory system develops through five distinct, yet overlapping phases: *embryonic*, *pseudoglandular*, *canalicular*, *saccular*, and *alveolar* [7]. While a full review of the embryology is not necessary for the understanding of neonatal respiratory care, it is important to note that each particular phase leads to unique respiratory difficulties and opportunities. Lung growth begins in the third week of gestation during the *embryonic* phase, with a small growth of diverticulum from the ventral wall of the foregut. This is often referred to as the primitive respiratory diverticulum or primitive lung bud [7]. Three rounds of branching and division also occur during this phase, leading to a left & right half as well as the formation of multiple tertiary bronchi. The vascular components of the respiratory system also begin their development during this phase. The *pseudoglandular* phase occurs from weeks 5–17, and this time period is notable for the completion of all bronchial divisions as well as formation of cilia and cartilage [8]. After this phase, any further lung growth is simply by the elongation, widening and hypertrophy of existing tissue. The *canalicular* phase is particularly important, as it encompasses 16–26 weeks of development and includes neonates of periviable gestational ages (ie, around 23 weeks gestation). Here, the earliest capillary beds begin to form, and areas of gas exchange start to develop. Many of the overlying epithelial cells also begin to thin out and improve the air-blood interface, further enhancing regions of gas exchange. More importantly, these cells also start to differentiate into type I pneumocytes that help form and stabilize the alveoli. Type II pneumocytes also start to appear, and these cells are vitally important in the production of endogenous surfactant [7, 8]. The canalicular stage is the earliest gestational age at which interventions can be provided. The *saccular* phase occurs from weeks 24–38 and leads to further development of alveolar ducts and conducting airways. Mucous and cilated cell growth also increases. Surfactant synthesis continues to improve, but overall production compared to full-term infants remains low [9]. This time period encompasses the bulk of premature infants, including those that are "late preterm." The relative structural immaturity coupled with insufficient (and often ineffective) surfactant production explains the need for respiratory support in this age group, even in infants born beyond 34 weeks gestation. Finally, the *alveolar* phase occurs from about 36 weeks – 8 years of age. This final stage is mainly characterized by further development of alveolar units, thinning of the air-blood interface, increased surface area for gas exchange, and increased numbers of type II pneumocytes, leading to enhanced synthesis of surfactant [7].

Throughout fetal development, fetal lung fluid is vital in the growth of normal lung structure. Fetal lung fluid is an isotonic fluid secreted by epithelial cells that helps promote growth and development. It is low in protein and high in chloride ions. Combined with contractions of fetal airway smooth muscle and fetal breathing in utero, these processes help promote the normal developmental process of lung growth. Fluid clearance is a process initiated by various labor mechanisms, and this also presents an area for maladaptation and one etiology of respiratory distress after birth [10].

Lung function in neonates, especially those born prematurely, is altered for a number of reasons. Structural issues include poorly developed lung parenchyma, airways and a highly elastic chest wall, and surfactant deficiency complicates these issues. This results in dramatic changes in normal lung mechanics and physiology, manifested by an overall state of abnormally decreased compliance, low functional residual capacity (FRC), and increased respiratory effort by the neonate [8]. This is further compounded by deranged gas exchange. If undertreated, each of these mechanisms may combine to cause respiratory failure. Antenatal steroids improve some of the structural and biochemical derangements, but post-natally the clinician must provide the correct level of respiratory support and surfactant when appropriate. The goal, as we will discuss, is resolve the skewed lung mechanics towards a more normal physiologic state by re-establishing FRC and decreasing work of breathing.

Functional residual capacity (FRC) is defined as the volume of air remaining in the lungs after a normal passive exhalation [8]. In most term, healthy neonates, this figure is typically about 20–30 mL/kg. To understand the significance of FRC in the management of neonatal respiratory care, it is important to understand normal transitional events in early postnatal life. During gestation, the developing fetus is entirely dependent on the placenta for gas exchange. This in-utero circulatory pattern consists of very limited pulmonary blood flow with intracardiac shunts in place to allow for adequate flow of blood to vital organs. The approximate oxygen saturation in a term fetus prior to delivery is about 60% [2]. When labor is initiated, epithelial lung cells halt their production of fetal lung fluid and begin to actively absorb it back into circulation. This process is triggered by thyroid hormone, glucocorticoids and epinephrine working in combination to change epithelial cells from chloride secreting to sodium reabsorption [11]. With the neonate's first spontaneous breaths, the lungs inflate and there is an increase in pulmonary arterial pO2 as well as activation of stretch receptors. This process, in conjunction with production of endogenous nitric oxide, dramatically reduces pulmonary vascular resistance [2]. As pulmonary vascular resistance continues to decrease, more pulmonary blood flow is established and oxygen saturations steadily increase to normal postnatal levels. The intra-cardiac shunts at the level of the ductus arteriosus and foramen ovale close due to increasing arterial oxygen content and increasing systemic vascular resistance from clamping of the umbilical cord, respectively. This process results in physiologic changes that can be witnessed in real time, as most healthy term neonates will obtain oxygen saturations greater than 90% by about 10 minutes of life.

For gas exchange to properly occur after birth, there must be an immediate interface between environmental oxygen and pulmonary blood flow at the alveolar-capillary level. Ventilation (V) and perfusion (Q) ratios reflect this physiologic state, and there are a number of ways that this process can be deranged. To allow for a normal VQ matching, there must be both an adequate alveolar gas volume and normal FRC [7]. If adequately sustained, either due to spontaneous respirations or assisted ventilation, FRC serves as an intrapulmonary pool of oxygen. Preterm infants and ill term infants are prone to a low FRC. This may lead to decreased compliance, increased airway resistance, increased work of breathing, increased pulmonary vascular resistance, hypoxemia, atelectasis, and impaired gas exchange [8]. Conversely, too much FRC from overinflation can also have negative effects and may lead to lung injury, air leaks and decreased cardiac output. Positive distending pressure is therefore critical in recruiting collapsed alveoli and establishing optimal FRC in neonates that cannot achieve it spontaneously (**Figure 1**).

Specific mechanical and physical properties of the lung also play an important role in neonatal respiratory care. The elasticity of a system refers to the property of matter such that a system will tend to return to its original position when all external forces are abated [8]. In the neonate, the elastic properties of the lung refer to not just the parenchyma, but also the air exchange spaces, muscle, connective tissue and vasculature. In addition, there is also a recoil effect from surface tension in the alveoli, which is artificially increased with impaired surfactant production. Lastly, there are opposing elastic forces that may be provide by the chest wall to assist with lung expansion and air entry. All of these elastic forces form a complex, interdependent balance that may determine FRC [8].

The pressure required to inflate a lung is directly proportional to the volume of inflation – this is often referred to as Hooke's Law [7]. While this relationship is often seen as an extension of the elastic properties of the lung, it brings us to our next biophysical property of respiratory physiology. The compliance of a lung is strictly defined as the change in lung volume due to a change in distending pressure during normal breathing, expressed as a ratio [8]. This is an extension of Hooke's Law. Compliance may be further divided into static and dynamic compliance. Static compliance refers to the tendency of the lung to recoil to its original dimensions after a known volume of pressure is applied and then removed [2]. Dynamic compliance, on the other hand, is measured during spontaneous breathing and refers to the change in pressure from the end of exhalation to the end of inspiration for a given volume. It reflects both the intrinsic elastic and resistive properties of the lung [2]. The compliance of a given respiratory system includes both the lung and the chest wall. In neonates, the chest wall is primarily made up of cartilage and thus is a high compliance system. Conversely, the compliance of the

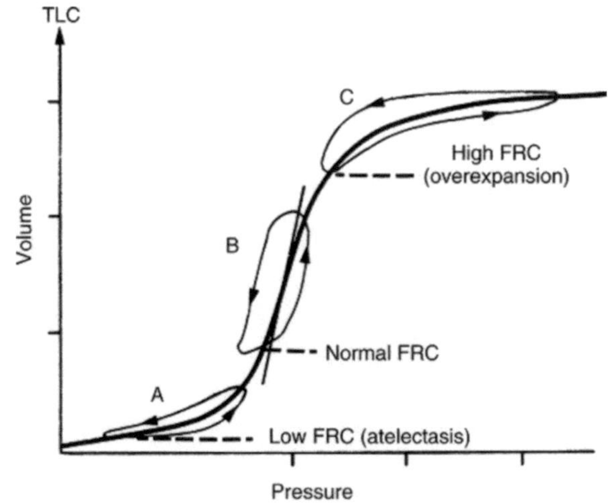

Figure 1. Compliance curve demonstrating different states of FRC. Area A represents poor lung volumes or collapse, where area C represents over distension of the lung. Area B demonstrates optimal lung volumes in which normal physiological FRC is maintained. Image used with permission by Elsevier Books, Inc.

lung is relatively low given surfactant deficiency and decreased alveolar radius, especially in premature infants [7]. This is a problematic scenario, as the balance of forces thereby is tilted towards lung collapse. This also negatively impacts FRC. Neonates respond by augmenting their FRC by increasing expiratory resistance through laryngeal abduction, clinically manifested as "grunting" [7]. Additionally, the higher respiratory rates seen in infants in low-compliant states creates relative gas trapping that helps slightly improve FRC [2]. The definitive treatment, however, is to deliver optimal PEEP via CPAP or another non-invasive modality to avoid atelectotrauma and to re-establish and sustain FRC (**Figure 2**).

The resistance to gas flow in a closed respiratory system is an important determinant of respiratory mechanics in neonates. Resistance is the direct result of friction, and can be defined as either viscous or airway resistance [2]. Viscous resistance refers to the resistance encountered by tissue elements as they touch and move past one another. Airway resistance refers to the resistance that occurs between moving gas molecules and between these molecules and the walls of the respiratory system [2]. Airway resistance makes up the majority of total resistance in a neonate. It is determined by the relationship between the velocity of gas flow, length of the airways, viscosity of the gas, and the diameter of the conducting airways. For laminar flow where all gas molecules move in an orderly fashion perfectly parallel to the walls of the airway, resistance is described by Poiseuille's law. This states that resistance is directly proportional to the product of the tube length and gas viscosity, and inversely proportional the airway radius to the fourth power [2]. Thus airway diameter is the critical determinant

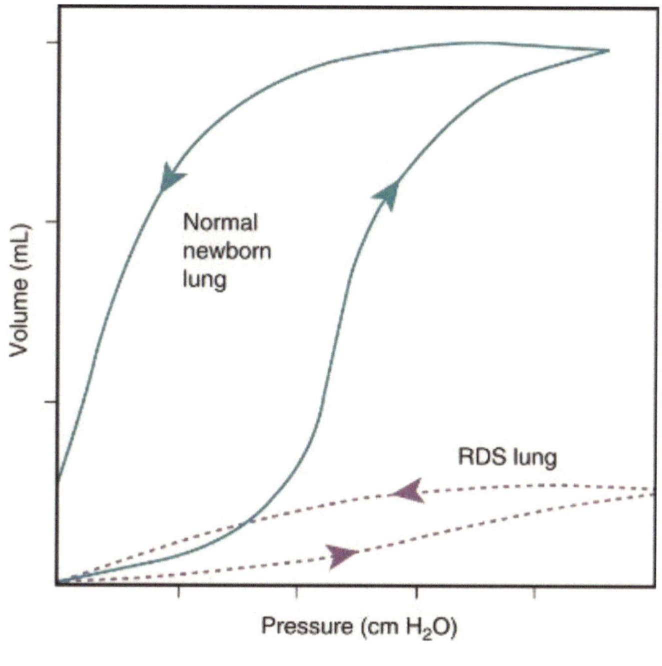

Figure 2. Comparison of compliance curves between a normal neonate (solid line) versus that of a neonate with RDS (dotted line). Note the very little volume change for an applied pressure seen in the infant with RDS due to the lack of surfactant and poor alveolar stabilization. Image used with permission by Elsevier Books, Inc.

of airway resistance, as even small changes in airway radius will have exponential effects on resistance. This effect in neonates is especially exaggerated as they have narrow airways relative to adults.

There is an inverse, nonlinear relationship between airway resistance and lung volume. This is due to the fact that airway size increases as FRC increases, therefore decreasing the total resistance of the system [2]. The converse is also true: any pathologic state in which low lung volumes occur will increase the airway resistance of that system. This is another lung mechanical property that is affected by the FRC. That is, application of adequate PEEP via non-invasive ventilation will establish optimal FRC, increase airway size, and decrease airway resistance [2].

One final concept to explore is work of breathing. Clinically, this term refers to the signs of respiratory distress exhibited by a patient. This can be manifested by tachypnea, grunting, intercostal retractions, or nasal flaring. Mathematically, work of breathing can be quantified as the energy needed to overcome the existing elastic and resistive forces. More specifically, this can be defined as the product of the force exerted and the volume of air displaced [2]. About two-thirds of this energy expenditure is used to overcome the elastic forces of the respiratory system, while one-third is used to overcome resistance [2]. While most clinicians recognize that a neonate exhibiting increased work of breathing is at risk for respiratory deterioration, it is important to realize that increased energy expenditure also results in increased oxygen consumption [8]. It is apparent that work of breathing can be decreased by the application of positive pressure via CPAP or some other non-invasive modality – but how? Of all the respiratory muscles, the diaphragm carries the majority of the workload. Like most skeletal muscles, its ability to generate optimal force is related to its initial relaxed position and the length of muscle fibers at the beginning of contraction [2]. Delivering PEEP via CPAP will not only help better inflate the lungs, but move the diaphragm into a more optimal position for contraction. In addition, PEEP may prevent atelectasis and move the neonate to a more ideal position on the pressure-volume curve where either extreme in atelectasis or over-distended are avoided, and instead optimal FRC is achieved [2, 12]. Lastly, one major role of the nasopharynx and lining of the upper airway is to provide warmth and moisture to inspired air. Non-invasive ventilation replaces the warming and humidification process required by the neonate, and in turn this may reduce metabolic demand [13].

4. Interface devices for providing non-invasive ventilation

Since Gregory's initial description of CPAP *via* a head-box, the technology used to provide continuous distending pressure to neonates has greatly evolved, first with the introduction of binasal prongs. Subsequently, both Kattwinkel et al. and Caliumi-Pellegrini et al. described non-invasive devices in which binasal prongs were connected to a ventilator to provide both flow and pressure [2]. This approach remained standard for a number of years. While the latter parts of this chapter will focus on each of the specific non-invasive modalities themselves, there is a considerable amount of overlap in terms of using the interface devices.

Devices such as "head boxes" or negative pressure boxes are purely of historical interest and are no longer in clinical practice. Facial masks can be used to provide CPAP provided that the mask is attached to a flow-inflating bag or a T-piece resuscitator (for more precise pressures generated). This is a commonly used approach in the delivery room for initial stabilization of neonates, but rarely used in a prolonged manner. Nasal masks, on the other hand, are often used to provide long-term support to neonates receiving non-invasive ventilation. This is typically with variable-flow devices or SiPAP [8]. Nasal prongs, however, are the most popular and effective way to provide non-invasive ventilation. Neonates are obligate nasal breathers so prongs provide the most reliable way of delivering consistent distending pressure [8]. If the infant's mouth is open, however, a large leak of pressure may occur and the neonate will not receive prescribed distending pressure. This may be addressed by using a chin strap or pacifier to keep the mouth closed. One other area where leak and loss of pressure can occur is at the nares; it is vital for nasal prongs to be large enough to fill the space within the nares to prevent this, but at the same time not so wide that they injure the surrounding mucosa and tissues [2, 8]. Long, thin prongs are generally avoided as they may increase the resistance in the system and even minor secretions can lead to significant obstruction and increased work of breathing. Endotracheal tubes are sometimes cut and used as "nasopharyngeal prongs." This practice is less common given all the previously described advantages of shorter binasal prongs. In addition, a recent Cochrane review also suggested that binasal prongs are simply more effective [14]. While we will explore some of the complications associated with non-invasive ventilation later in the chapter, skin and nasal trauma is perhaps the most commonly encountered issue. Adequate skin care requires assiduous nursing care, and often skin barriers are applied.

The pressure delivered by CPAP is typically *via* a continuous or variable flow device. Continuous flow was the method originally used in the 1970s and 1980s, and historically relied on gas flow generated from a ventilator [2]. Continuous-flow CPAP is still used today, typically *via* bubble or water-seal CPAP; this will be described in detail later in this chapter. Two of the most commonly used binasal prongs in continuous-flow CPAP are the Hudson (Hudson Respiratory Care, Inc., Arlington Heights, Illinois, USA) and Inca (Ackrad Laboratories, Inc., Cranford, New Jersey, USA) prongs. Argyle prongs are also occasionally used, but have fallen out of favor [14]. Many of these binasal prongs are interchangeable with different modes of non-invasive support, including CPAP, SiPAP/BiPAP or even nasal intermittent positive pressure ventilation (NIPPV) via a ventilator [15]. There are scant comparative studies in the literature comparing one prong type to another [2] (**Figure 3**).

Nasal masks are another avenue of providing non-invasive ventilation. The mask itself is connected to the pressure generator, typically a variable-flow device. Many units alternate the use of nasal masks with prongs to help prevent nasal and mucosal trauma. As with prongs, leaks can decrease the amount of pressure delivered to the patient. Therefore a proper seal around the nose must be maintained at all times. Very little data exists about the safety and efficacy of nasal masks versus prongs, and there are currently no reported studies of using NIPPV via nasal mask [2, 15] (**Figure 4**).

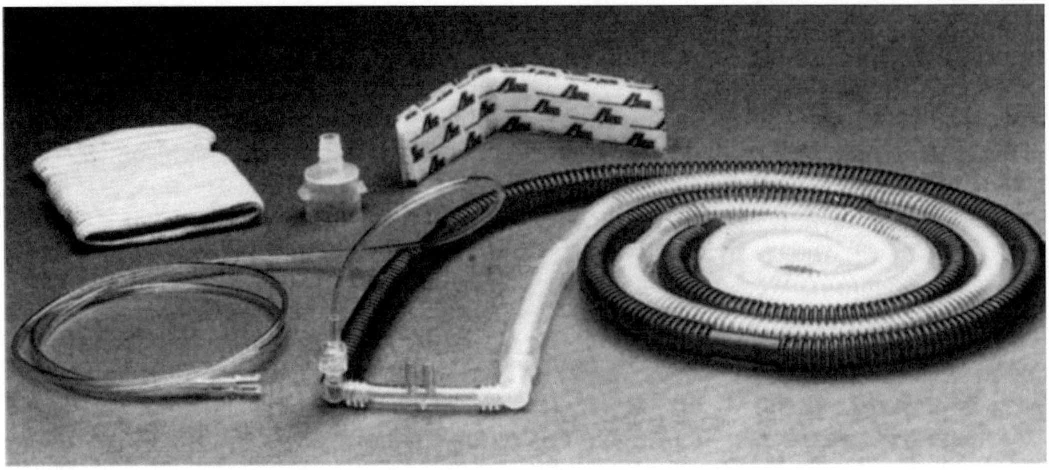

Figure 3. The Hudson NCPAP equipment very commonly used in many NICUs. Image used with permission by Elsevier Books, Inc.

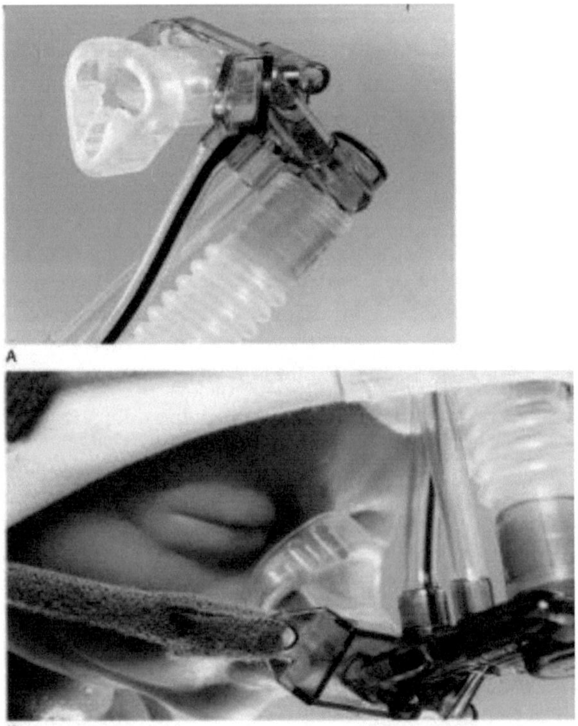

Figure 4. An example of a typical nasal mask used to deliver NCPAP with the infant flow driver device. Image used with permission by Elsevier Books, Inc.

While nasal cannulae (NC) are routinely used to provide supplemental oxygen, some distending pressure can be generated. The rate of gas flow, size of the cannulae, and degree of leak around the nares determine the amount of pressure generated [2]. Higher flow rates delivered with relatively large sized nasal cannulae is termed "high flow nasal cannulae" (HFNC). Often heated and humidified, the physiology of respiratory support provided by HFNC is different than CPAP. The primary concern with a HFNC system is that depending on the flow rate and degree of leak, very high, uncontrolled positive pressure may be delivered. Not all HFNC devices contain "pop-off" valves to prevent this. These concepts will be explored later in this chapter. Finally, the RAM Nasal Cannula (Neotech, Valencia, California, USA) was originally designed to provide supplemental oxygen, but is a versatile interface device [2]. It has been used in various forms of CPAP as well as NIPPV *via* a ventilator. While at its core it is essentially another short binasal prong, it is designed with larger bore tubing to help reduce resistance and dead space. It has gained widespread use in many NICUs for its relative ease of use [2]. Early anecdotal reports also suggested lower rates nasal trauma. Concerns regarding the RAM Nasal Cannula have to do with the long segment of narrow tubing from the circuit connector to the prongs, creating a great deal of resistance. This can potentially lead to a sizeable drop in pressure and also raises concern about whether the clinician can accurately assess if the patient is receiving the desired distending pressure. It is important to also note that the use of the RAM Nasal Cannula in providing non-invasive ventilation is currently considered off-label use, as it is only approved for providing supplemental oxygen at this time.

5. Nasal continuous positive airway pressure (NCPAP)

Continuous positive airway pressure (CPAP) is positive pressure applied to the airways of spontaneously breathing neonates. As previously discussed, the primary function of the respiratory system is to move ambient air into the lungs for gas exchange. Any factor that limits this basic physiology will predispose the neonate to respiratory failure [8]. The inability to establish and maintain adequate lung volumes is perhaps the biggest risk factor for compromise. Low lung volumes and the resulting atelectasis may result in ventilation-perfusion mismatch and intrapulmonary shunting of blood. Oxygenation is typically affected the most, and while carbon dioxide can generally diffuse across biological membranes easily, its removal can be hampered by a low lung-volume state. Other mechanisms that contribute to respiratory distress in neonates include: retained lung fluid and pulmonary edema, suboptimal FRC, unstable chest wall with high compliance, upper airway more prone to collapse, poor laryngeal tone, and surfactant deficiency [8].

5.1. Physiological benefits of CPAP

CPAP alleviates many of physiologic derangements by increasing mean airway pressure and distending the airways to establish and maintain optimal FRC. By stabilizing and opening terminal alveoli, surface area for gas exchange is enhanced, and ventilation-perfusion mismatching is reduced. CPAP also improves diaphragmatic contractility. In addition, CPAP decreases the range of different opening pressure gradients between different areas of the lung and helps homogenize the total delivered tidal ventilations [8]. By better distending the individual alveolar units, CPAP also reduces the pressure needed to overcome surface tension. Surfactant is better preserved on the alveolar surface, further preventing atelectasis and the resulting atelectotrauma. In addition, CPAP has been shown to reduce upper airway occlusion by increasing pharyngeal cross-sectional area and decreasing upper airway resistance [8]. Coupled with stabilization of the chest wall and improved compliance, CPAP also reduces work of breathing. Apnea of prematurity is a common issue for many neonates born before 35 weeks gestation. It is manifested by various episodes of apnea, bradycardia and oxygenation desaturation, or some combination of the three. While there is very limited evidence of CPAP being an effective treatment for apnea of prematurity, it is often clinically used in such a manner [2].

5.2. Methods of CPAP delivery

The pressure delivered via CPAP is either via a continuous flow or variable flow device. One of the most common methods of providing continuous-flow CPAP is what is referred to as bubble or water-seal CPAP [2]. Blended gas is first heated and humidified, then delivered to the neonate, typically *via* binasal prongs or a nasal mask. The distal end of the expiratory tubing is submerged in either 0.25% acetic acid or sterile water to a specific depth; this depth determines the level of CPAP generated [2]. The bubbles from the exhalation limb produce observable chest vibrations that could potentially enhance gas exchange. Furthermore, the applied gas flow rate to the CPAP device affects the degree of bubbling, suggesting that there may be a low-amplitude, high-frequency oscillatory effect to the lungs [13]. Initial studies that reported these findings, however, were using bubble CPAP delivered via a nasopharyngeal tube and not binasal prongs [2]. More studies are needed to determine if there exists an oscillatory waveform that enhances ventilation while on bubble CPAP.

Variable-flow CPAP has been in use since 1995 and was originally developed by Moa et al. to help reduce neonatal work of breathing [2]. These devices use dual injector jets directed towards each nasal prong to establish a constant airway pressure. In addition, when the neonate makes a spontaneous expiration, there is a "fluidic flip" in which the flow of gas is reversed and allowed to exit via the expiratory limb of the device. This phenomenon is enhanced due to the Coanda effect, in which gas tends to follow a curved surface [2]. The two most common variable-flow devices currently available are the Infant Flow (Cardinal Health, Dublin, Ohio, USA) and the Arabella system (Hamilton Medical, Reno, Nevada, USA). Some studies have indeed demonstrated less work of breathing and better synchrony in neonates on variable-flow devices compared to bubble CPAP. Others have found similar rates of extubation failure after randomization to either bubble CPAP or variable-flow CPAP following extubation from mechanical ventilation [2]. Despite these differences in the literature, there is no definitive evidence to suggest one mode of CPAP is superior. Many of these studies were done with neonates of various gestational ages and weights, which may confound the results further. Clearly, the clinician must be familiar with the device(s) available to them in their particular units and to be comfortable with their management.

5.3. Clinical management of CPAP

Determining the optimal CPAP level should be individualized to each neonate's underlying pathophysiology and should be aimed to obtain optimal without over-distention. This target may change based on the neonate's disease course and postnatal age. The use of correctly sized binasal prongs with a chinstrap or pacifier to keep the mouth closed (if needed) is important to minimize any loss of pressure. Immediately after birth, most neonates of all gestational are started on a level of 5 or 6 cm H_2O, with escalation to 8–10 cm H_2O as needed [2, 8]. There is limited evidence, however, to suggest a singular approach to initiating or changing the CPAP level. Again, these decisions should be driven by the underlying pathophysiology and supported by clinical and laboratory measures when necessary. Many institutions have their own specific guidelines and goals, especially when caring for the very low birthweight or extremely low birthweight infant. In general, the CPAP level is deemed appropriate when the neonate's oxygenation and ventilation are satisfactory, the chest radiograph is optimally inflated, work of breathing is minimal, and the neonate is otherwise hemodynamically stable. When the CPAP level is too high, one may see signs of over-distention on the chest radiograph manifested by a flattened diaphragm or small heart size. Gas exchange may be worsened and, in severe cases, over-distention can reduce cardiac output leading to tachycardia and hypotension [8].

Weaning the neonate off CPAP is another area that should be driven by the underlying physiology and any continued need for respiratory support. This is typically possible when the neonate is requiring little to no supplemental oxygen, work of breathing is negligible, and there are few episodes of apnea, bradycardia, and desaturation [8]. While some institutions wean the CPAP level during this time, other institutions do not. An alternative method of weaning CPAP consists of "sprinting" the neonate off CPAP support for a period of time, which gradually increases until off entirely. This is not well studied and this method of "sprinting" may actually lead to CPAP weaning failure and may prolong the length of time ultimately spent on CPAP [8]. Additional questions include at what postnatal age to consider removal of CPAP, and what level of support (if any) should the neonate be transitioned to. The duration of CPAP is often driven by the neonate's gestational age even in the absence of significant lung disease, as very preterm infants often benefit from longer use of CPAP while their chest walls mature and offset the elastic recoil of the lungs [8]. While this may vary from one institution to another, typical goals for removing an extremely preterm neonate from CPAP are around 32–34 weeks postmenstrual age, when appropriate goals are achieved (ie, no work of breathing and/or minimal supplemental oxygen requirement, etc). When discontinuing CPAP, the neonate can either be taken directly to room air or transitioned to a lesser mode of support (typically some form of nasal cannula). Again, much of this decision-making is driven by the current lung disease (if any) being treated at the time, as well as any other factors that may predispose the neonate to continued need for respiratory support. For example, the neonate that is otherwise stable on a fairly low CPAP level, has no oxygen requirement, and is growing well can reasonably be taken to room air as the initial attempt at discontinuing CPAP. The neonate that still has a minimal oxygen requirement but otherwise meets other criteria for coming off CPAP can be taken to a nasal cannula.

5.4. BiPAP and SiPAP

Bilevel CPAP (BiPAP) or sigh intermittent positive airway pressure (SiPAP) has been marketed as a means of delivering alternating levels of distending pressure. Both are typically used with the Infant Flow driver and can alternate between a lower and higher CPAP pressure throughout the respiratory cycle; some ventilators can provide this mode as well [2]. This method of support is not synchronized (synchrony is currently only available in Europe and Canada), and the neonate breathes spontaneously at both levels of support. This potentially creates two distinct FRCs [16]. The CPAP levels cycle at a specific rate. The higher pressure level is delivered during "inspiration", with typical values of 8–10 cm H_2O, but sometimes as high as 15 cm H_2O if using a patient triggered BiPAP device. Most SiPAP devices, on the other hand, will have a "sigh" pop-off that will prevent inspiratory PEEP from exceeding 10 cm H_2O. During "expiration", the neonate will breathe the lower pressure level, with typical values set at 4–6 cm H_2O. A higher "inspiratory time" is typically used, with some authors suggested as high as 1 second [8]. Lista et al. compared outcomes in preterm neonates with RDS that were initially supported with CPAP versus SiPAP [16]. They found that infants supported with SiPAP had a shorter duration of mechanical ventilation overall, needed less oxygen, and were discharged home sooner. A caveat of these studies is that it can be difficult to compare the actually distending mean airway pressure delivered between CPAP and BiPAP/SiPAP. The latter, with alternating levels of pressure, will typically generate a pressure that is 2–3 cm H_2O higher than CPAP [2]. It is quite possible that it is this higher overall level of pressure in addition to the cyclical tidal volumes delivered that result in benefit to the infant. A recent study in 2016 by Victor et al. aimed to compare the use of CPAP and BiPAP in infants born before 30 weeks' gestation and less than two weeks old using equivalent mean airway pressures [17]. They did not find any difference in extubation failures between the two groups, nor did they find any difference in total duration of mechanical ventilation, oxygen requirement at 28 days & 36 weeks corrected, or length of hospitalization.

6. Humidified high flow nasal cannula (HHFNC)

HHFNC use rapidly expanded in NICUs since 2005. The two major commercially available devices are Vapotherm (Exeter, New Hampshire, USA) and Fisher & Paykel (Auckland, New Zealand) [2]. While most clinicians refer to this technology as "HFNC," the delivered air undergoes a heating and humidification process. Traditional nasal cannula was limited to flow rates of 2 lpm of either 100% or blended oxygen for neaontes [13]. Higher rates of flow often caused significant drying of the airway mucosa, leading to irritation and mucosal trauma. The new HFNC systems create nearly 100%, allowing clinicians to use higher flow rates. This can vary from one institution to another. Some centers will use flow rates of up to 4 lpm, while others use rates as high as 8 lpm. Many of the same physiological benefits seen with the use of CPAP can be extrapolated to the use of HHFNC, as the higher flow rates has been shown in some studies to provide comparable distending pressure [2]. These benefits include improved pharyngeal tone, nasopharyngeal deadspace washout, decreased work of breathing, and maintenance of FRC [13]. The primary concern with the use of HHFNC is that it can potentially deliver unpredictable, uncontrolled and widely variable levels of distending pressure. Some studies using esophageal probes have measured the pressure delivered by HHFNC; this level is a determined not only by the flow rate delivered, but also the weight of the neonate and the size of the cannulae [2]. Neither of the two commercially available HHFNC devices are capable of measuring the level of pressure provided. They do, however, have an internal pressure-limiting mechanism as a safety measure to prevent excessive pressures from reaching the patient [8]. Ultimately, though, there currently is no reliable way to calculate how much distending pressure is delivered. For that reason, it is vital that the nasal prongs selected allow for some leak around the nares so that extremely high pressures are avoided.

6.1. Clinical use of HHFNC

HHFNC has been tried in various domains of neonatal respiratory management, including as a means of avoiding extubation failure in premature neonates. There have been a handful of recent studies to look at this, and the general consensus seems to be that HHFNC was non-inferior to CPAP in terms of extubation failures [8]. The additional finding of less nasal and mucosal trauma was consistent across most of these studies. Overall, however, there is still insufficient evidence to suggest that HHFNC is equal or superior to CPAP in preventing extubation failure. Much of this has to do with wide variations in the previously mentioned study designs, use of different devices, and unknown severity of respiratory distress in enrolled patients [8]. These data are even more limited for extremely low birthweight infants or those born less than 28 weeks' gestation [13].

HHFNC has also been studied for treatment of apnea of prematurity and work of breathing. Saslow et al. (2006) evaluated the effects of CPAP and Vapotherm HFNC on work of breathing patterns in a crossover study of preterm infants requiring either support modality and weighing <2.0 kg at birth. They did not find any significant differences between the two groups [8]. Sreenan et al. (2011) also looked at stable premature infants in a crossover study of CPAP and HHFNC. They did not find any differences between the two modalities with respect to apnea, bradycardia, or desaturation events, oxygen requirement, or work of breathing [8]. This remains an area where success with HHFNC can certainly be achieved, but it is important to note that no definitive evidence exists to prove it is equally efficacious as CPAP.

6.2. Current best evidence regarding HHFNC use

In June 2015, an international group of experts met in Oxford, England to discuss the use of nasal high-flow therapy in neonatology. The goal of the meeting was to reach consensus among clinicians on how to best use and study HHFNC in neonates and to try to establish guidelines for its management [13]. At the time of their meeting, their review encompassed four current RCTs that involved over 1100 preterm infants [13]. The following is summary of the group's findings.

The Oxford group recommended that in general, HHFNC can be *considered* for most neonates in which CPAP would be used. This includes preterm infants with respiratory distress, increased work of breathing, or an oxygen requirement. Special consideration should be given to neonates with significant nasal trauma from CPAP use, as switching to HHFNC may allow the nares to heal [13]. The same level of monitoring and nursing care provided to a neonate on CPAP should be applied to a neonate on HHFNC [13].

As previously mentioned, one of the major differences at the level of the nasal prongs between CPAP and HHFNC is the desired amount of leak. With HHFNC, there must be a moderate amount of leak around the nares to allow gas egress and to ensure that unpredictably high pressures do not occur. The group concluded that the prong dimensions be no greater than 50% of the diameter of the nares, and that the gas flow via HHFNC be heated between 34 and 37 degrees C [13]. Furthermore, the actual cannulae used should be per manufacturer recommendations, and components from different systems should not be mixed.

Individual institutions may have their own particular guidelines, but the Oxford meeting recommends starting with flows of 4–6 lpm for most preterm infants. Lower flow rates of 2–3 lpm may be acceptable for larger neonates closer to or at term [13]. A maximum flow rate of 8 lpm is recommended, and only in response to increased work of breathing or higher oxygen requirements. Escalation from HHFNC to a different support modality should be considered in cases of increased work of breathing, increased apnea, or oxygen requirements greater than 50% [13]. Weaning the flow rate can be considered once the neonate is stable for about 24 hours and on 30% or less oxygen, with one recommended approach of weaning the flow rate by 1 lpm every 12 hours as tolerated. Again, institutions may have their own weaning protocols. Discontinuing HHFNC can be considered once flow rates of 2–4 lpm are achieved, as 2 lpm is actually the lowest most devices will sustain, and the benefits of rates less than 3 lpm are actually unclear at this point [13].

6.3. Summary

A growing body of evidence seems to suggest that HHFNC is fairly safe and efficacious in supporting many preterm infants, however no definitive evidence exists. Flow rates of 2–8 lpm are generally acceptable, with careful attention to prong size and adherence to all manufacturer recommendations. Clearly, however, more research is needed. Specifically, more studies are needed to evaluate the use of HHFNC in extremely low birth weight infants and those born less than 27 weeks' gestation, as well as the potential use of HHFNC in delivery room resuscitation and during neonatal transport [13]. *This is one specific age group in which the evidence still overwhelmingly supports the use of CPAP as the initial mode of support.* More studies are also needed to compare different HHFNC devices, types of cannulas, and true flow rate recommendations based on weight and gestational age. Finally, the Oxford group strongly recommends that each institution devise and adhere to their own agreed-upon guidelines so that a standardized approach to the use of HHFNC can be applied and subsequently studied.

7. Nasal intermittent positive pressure ventilation (NIPPV)

Nasal intermittent mandatory ventilation (NIMV), also known as nasal intermittent positive pressure ventilation (NIPPV), refers to ventilation provided via a conventional ventilator in a non-invasive fashion. This is usually administered *via* short binasal prongs, the RAM Nasal Cannula, or a nasal mask [2, 8]. Depending on the type of ventilator and settings used, NIPPV is designed to deliver positive pressure throughout the respiratory cycle with defined, intermittent increases in pressure, often in synchrony with respiratory efforts [8]. This method of respiratory support was initially described in the early 1970s when *via* time-cycled inflations using a ventilator with an oronasal mask [2]. In the 1980s, more than 50% of the level III NICUs in Canada were consistently using this method of respiratory support. Shortly after, it fell out of favor due to reports of facial neurological injuries and gastrointestinal perforations; subsequent studies regarding the use of NIPPV in neonates have not reported higher rates of these complications [2, 13]. Of note, nasal high-frequency ventilation (NHFV) is also described in the literature and is increasingly common in some centers in Europe. Given its relative new nature and lack of extensive comparative studies, it will not be discussed here.

7.1. Benefits of NIPPV

The physiological benefits of NIPPV are similar to other modes of positive pressure delivery. Specifically, NIPPV will expand the lung and recruit terminal alveoli, increase FRC, prevent atelectasis and atelectotrauma, and improve ventilation-perfusion mismatches [8, 18]. In addition, the positive pressure delivered helps splint the upper airways, improves laryngeal tone, and stabilizes the highly compliant neonatal chest wall. Synchronized NIPPV, or sNIPPV, has been shown in several studies to deliver higher tidal volumes than CPAP or non-synchronized NIPPV [13, 18]. In addition, all forms of NIPPV deliver additional positive pressure breaths, further increasing mean airway pressure. This in turn helps to further improve tidal volumes and reduces thoraco-abdominal asynchrony (especially true with sNIPPV), which has may reduce work of breathing and improve pulmonary mechanics [8]. Animal studies have also shown that the intermittent distending pressure above PEEP that NIPPV provides can more effectively recruit the lung than CPAP alone, leading to further improvements in FRC [13].

NIPPV has been studied in three major domains: preventing extubation failures, treating apnea of prematurity, and as the primary mode of treating respiratory distress in premature neonates. As of 2015, there have been ten randomized controlled trials comparing NIPPV with CPAP after extubation in premature infants. Friedlich et al. were the first to publish a study comparing CPAP with sNIPPV, and demonstrated that sNIPPV reduced extubation failures significantly [19]. In 2017, a Cochrane meta-analysis of these trials demonstrated a reduction in extubation failure (NNT = 4), but the studies included various NIPPV devices with a mix of synchrony versus asynchrony [8]. Furthermore, there was variability in the definition of extubation success. Despite these *caveats*, the conclusion from the review was that NIPPV may reduce extubation failure within 48 hours to one week after extubation more effectively than CPAP. No effect, however, was seen on chronic lung disease or mortality [18].

For treatment of apnea of prematurity, there are three studies comparing CPAP with NIPPV. The evidence is conflicting and there is no current recommendation whether NIPPV is superior to CPAP [8, 13]. A total of eight studies with 850 patients have looked at NIPPV as the primary mode of initial ventilation in premature neonates with respiratory distress syndrome, with the primary outcome being failure of non-invasive support and the need for intubation. The studies included different devices with mixed populations. Furthermore, some studies allowed the use of surfactant while others did not. As one might imagine, the results were mixed, with six of the trials essentially finding no difference between the two respiratory modalities [8]. As mentioned above, the strongest evidence in this area as demonstrated by the 2017 Cochrane review appears to be the use of NIPPV to prevent extubation failure when used immediately after extubation [18].

7.2. Typical NIPPV settings

As with every mode of respiratory support, the settings applied to any particular neonate should be based on the particular device used and the underlying pathophysiology. Initial settings on NIPPV are typically similar to those of a mechanical ventilator, with two exceptions, applied peak inspiratory pressure (PIP) and inspiratory time (Ti). Higher PIP is often necessary as pressure is delivered via a nasal interface and pressure is attenuated prior to delivery to the lungs. Therefore, NIPPV PIP is typically started about 2–4 cm H_2O higher than that normally used for mechanical ventilation *via* an endotracheal tube [8]. This is then adjusted based on adequate chest rise and blood gas measurements. For similar reasons, slightly higher inspiratory times of 0.4–0.5 seconds are also typical, as breaths delivered nasally have more resistance to overcome versus those delivered via an endotracheal tube.

Weaning from conventional ventilator to NIPPV should be done according to the same general recommendations as for any other mode. The goal should be well inflated lungs with an adequate FRC and minimal work of breathing. Settings on NIPPV are typically similar to prior settings on mechanical ventilation at the time of extubation. While this will differ from one institution to the next, this typically consists of rates below 25 breaths/min, a PIP of less than 20 cm H_2O, and an oxygen requirement of less than 30–35%. PEEP can be variable depending on oxygen requirement and need for lung expansion, but ideally will be 6 cm H_2O or less [8].

8. Summary

Although the means of delivering non-invasive respiratory support are widely variable, with numerous interfaces, devices and modes, the underlying goal is the same for all. Each baby's physiology should be assessed and non-invasive respiratory support must be tailored to resolve the most important underlying pathophysiology. When properly supported, babies should be well oxygenated, with minimal work of breathing, infrequent apnea, and a stable respiratory status.

Acknowledgements

I would like to thank my colleagues, Drs. Schlegel and Shepherd, for all their support and guidance in undertaking this endeavor. Furthermore, I want to recognize all of the neonatal nurse practitioners, nurses, respiratory therapists, pharmacists, nutritionists, and occupational/physical therapists that work so tirelessly so that we can provide the best care for our most vulnerable patients.

Author details

Omid Fathi*, Amy Brown Schlegel and Edward G. Shepherd

*Address all correspondence to: omid.fathi@nationwidechildrens.org

Assistant Professor of Clinical Pediatrics, Division of Neonatology, Nationwide Children's Hospital & The Ohio State College of Medicine, Columbus, OH, USA

References

[1] Gregory GA et al. Treatment of the idiopathic respiratory-distress syndrome with continuous positive airway pressure. The New England Journal of Medicine. 1971;**284**:1333-1340

[2] Goldsmith Jay P, Karotkin E, Keszler M, Suresh G, editors. Assisted Ventilation of the Neonate: An Evidence-Based Approach to Newborn Respiratory Care. 6th ed. Philadelphia: Elsevier; 2017 500 p

[3] Berger TM, Fontana M, Stocker M. The journey towards lung protective respiratory support in preterm neonates. Neonatology. 2013;**104**:265-274. DOI: 10.1159/000354419

[4] Avery ME, Mead J. Surface properties in relation to atelectasis and hyaline membrane disease. AMA J Dis Child. 1959;**97**:517-523

[5] Northway WH, Rosan R, Porter DY. Pulmonary disease following respirator therapy of hyaline-membrane disease: Bronchopulmonary dysplasia. The New England Journal of Medicine. 1967;**276**:357-368

[6] Avery ME, Tooley WH, Keller JB, Hurd SS, Bryan MH, Cotton RB, et al. Is chronic lung disease in low birth weight infants preventable? Pediatrics. 1987;**79**:26-30

[7] Davis RP, Mychaliska GB. Neonatal pulmonary physiology. Seminars in Pediatric Surgery. 2013 Nov;**22**(4):179-184. DOI: 10.1053/j.sempedsurg.2013.10.005

[8] Donn SM, Sinha SK, editors. Manual of Neonatal Respiratory Care. 4th ed. Cham, Switzerland: Springer International Publishing AG; 2017. 820 p. DOI: 10.1007/978-3-319-39839-6

[9] McBride W. Congenital lesions of the lung. NeoReviews. 2016;**17**(5):e263-e270. DOI: 10.1542/neo.17-5-e263

[10] Cullen AB, Wolfson MR, Shaffer TH. The maturation of airway structure and function. NeoReviews. 2002;**3**:e125-e130. DOI: 10.1542/neo.3-7-e125

[11] Jain L, Eaton DC. Physiology of fetal lung fluid clearance and the effect of labor. Seminars in Perinatology. 2006 Feb;**30**(1):34-43. DOI: 10.1053/j.semperi.2006.01.006

[12] Alexiou S, Panitch HB. Physiology of non-invasive respiratory support. Seminars in Fetal & Neonatal Medicine. 2016 Jun;**21**(3):174-180. DOI: 10.1016/j.siny.2016.02.007

[13] Yoder BA, Kirpalani H, editors. Non-Invasive Ventilation, an Issue of. Clinics in Perinatology. 1st ed. Philadelpha, PA: Elsevier; 2016 200 p

[14] De Paoli AG, Davis PG, Faber B, Morley CJ. Devices and pressure sources for administration of nasal continuous positive airway pressure (NCPAP) in preterm neonates. Cochrane Database of Systematic Reviews. 2008 Jan;**23**(1):CD002977. DOI: 10.1002/14651858.CD002977.pub2

[15] Owen LS, Manley BJ. Nasal intermittent positive pressure ventilation in preterm infants: Equipment, evidence, and synchronization. Seminars in Fetal & Neonatal Medicine. 2016 Jun;**21**(3):146-153. DOI: 10.1016/j.siny.2016.01.003

[16] Salvo V, Lista G, et al. Noninvasive ventilation strategies for early treatment of RDS in preterm infants: An RCT. Pediatrics. 2015 Mar;**135**(3):444-451. DOI: 10.1542/peds.2014-0895

[17] Victor S, Roberts SA, et al. Biphasic positive airway pressure of continuous positive airway pressure: A randomized trial. Pediatrics. 2016;**138**(2). DOI: 10.1542/peds.2015-4095

[18] Lemyre B, Davis PG, De Paoli AG, Kirpalani H. Nasal intermittent positive pressure ventilation (NIPPV) versus nasal continuous positive airway pressure (NCPAP) for preterm neonates after extubation. Cochrane Database of Systematic Reviews. 2017 Feb:1-75. DOI: 10.1002/14651858.CD003212.pub3

[19] Ramanathan R. Nasal respiratory support through the nares: Its time has come. Journal of Perinatology. 2010 Oct;**30**:S67-S72. DOI: 10.1038/jp.2010.99

Chapter 6

Open-Circuit Mouthpiece Ventilation: Indications, Evidence and Practicalities

Michalis Agrafiotis, Konstantina Nikolaou,
Dimitra Siopi and Diamantis Chloros

Additional information is available at the end of the chapter

http://dx.doi.org/10.5772/intechopen.73243

Abstract

Open-circuit mouthpiece ventilation (MPV) is a method of noninvasive ventilation, which can be used to provide full-time support, induce lung volume recruitment, increase cough efficacy, defer tracheostomy and possibly improve survival and quality of life in advanced-stage neuromuscular patients. MPV might also be applicable to other chronic respiratory diseases as well as in acute exacerbations of chronic obstructive pulmonary disease and can also be employed for the extubation of unweanable neuromuscular patients. A candidate for MPV should be able to rotate his neck adequately, grab the mouthpiece with his lips and maintain sufficient control of the upper airway muscles. MPV is usually provided in the volume assisted-controlled mode with a tidal volume between 0.7 and 1.5 L, zero PEEP and backup rate set to the lower allowed value, allowing the patient to define his own ventilatory pattern. The "low pressure" and "apnea" alarm should be switched off, if possible, or special setting adjustments should be used to prevent their activation. Comprehensive patient training and dedicated nursing time are important for the application of MPV. MPV is considered a safe method for the majority of the patients, but accidental mouthpiece loss is an important concern.

Keywords: noninvasive ventilation, tracheostomy, Duchenne muscular dystrophy, amyotrophic lateral sclerosis, home ventilation

1. Introduction: rationale for mouthpiece ventilation

Mouthpiece ventilation (MPV) is a unique method of respiratory support specifically intended to provide full-time ventilatory assistance mainly to patients with chronic ventilatory failure and limited or no ventilator-free breathing time [1–3]. Together with negative pressure ventilation, MPV is probably one of the oldest methods of noninvasive ventilatory support since it was initially employed as an alternative to tracheostomy by poliomyelitis survivors 60 years ago [3]. However, it was the pioneering work of a few investigators over the last three decades, which popularized the use of MPV for the management of chronic ventilatory failure, and since 2013, several MPV modes have been incorporated into modern home ventilators [3, 4–10].

The main indication of MPV is the provision of full-time ventilatory support for patients with chronic progressive neuromuscular diseases (NMD). Many NMDs cause respiratory disease by involving inspiratory, expiratory and upper airway muscles, leading to sleep disordered breathing, reduced respiratory pump efficiency and weak cough [11, 12]. From the respiratory physician's point of view, the most characteristic pathophysiologic trait of these NMDs is chronic alveolar hypoventilation which appears initially during the rapid eye movement sleep stage and extends eventually throughout all sleep stages before manifesting during daytime [13]. At advanced disease stages cough function is also severely impaired predisposing to respiratory infections and atelectasis [11, 12]. The institution of noninvasive positive pressure ventilation (NIV) for the support of the feeble respiratory muscles at the early stage of nocturnal hypoventilation is the mainstay of management of these patients and has been shown to improve survival, quality of sleep and quality of life [14–19]. However, as disease progresses and respiratory muscles continue to weaken, ventilatory requirements extend into the daytime. For patients with limited or no ventilator-free breathing time (e.g. ventilator use for > 16 or 20 hours per day), many practitioners would suggest transition to invasive ventilation via tracheostomy [20]. Importantly, an additional role of tracheostomy is the facilitation of secretion clearance given that at advanced disease stages cough flows are invariably reduced [11, 12]. In a European survey involving patients managed with home ventilation, patients with NMDs were the most likely to receive ventilatory support for a prolonged period (>6 years) and to have undergone tracheostomy procedures [21]. Nevertheless, long-term tracheostomies have been associated with several disadvantages including loss of voice, tube-related injuries, increased care-giver burden and disturbed self-image [2, 3, 9]. Although most patients would show preference toward a continued noninvasive mode of management [6, 22], standard nasal or oronasal masks are not suitable for this task since they commonly cause difficulties in eating, drinking and speech, sense of claustrophobia, limited field of vision, impaired social interaction and pressure lesions [1–3].

An alternative method for continuous noninvasive ventilator support is based on the 24 hour use of MPV or the combination of MPV during the daytime with nocturnal nasal or oronasal mask ventilation (MV). This method is complemented by ancillary strategies of which the most important are the "air-stacking" maneuver and the glossopharyngeal breathing (GPB) technique [1–3]. A good candidate for MPV should be able to rotate his neck and grab the mouthpiece with his lips and also maintain good control of his upper airway muscles (**Figure 1**) [10]. MPV is usually delivered via a home ventilator in the volume-assist-control mode (VAC) with the tidal volume (Vt) commonly set between 0.7 and 1.5 L (to correct for air leaks), zero PEEP and a back-up respiratory rate ideally set to zero [1–3]. Therefore, the patient has the ability to define his pattern of breathing according to his own ventilatory needs by taking as many breaths as he requires and by modifying the quantity of leak [8].

Volume-target MPV facilitates the application of the "air-stacking" maneuver, which is performed by teaching the patient to stack consecutive volumes of air delivered from the

http://dx.doi.org/10.5772/intechopen.73243

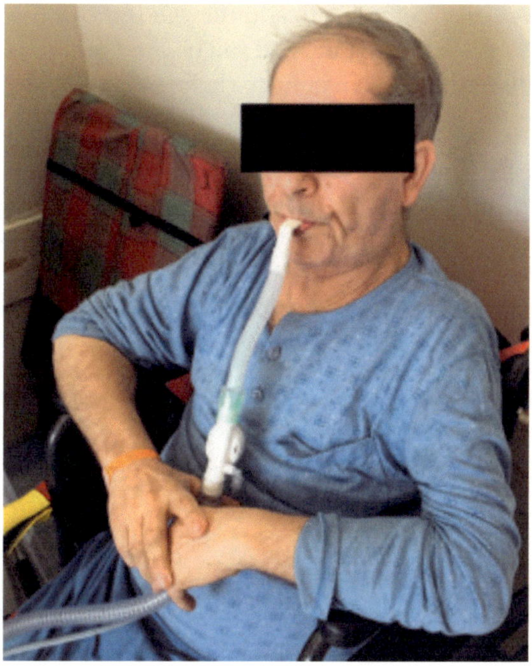

Figure 1. A patient with non-bulbar amyotrophic lateral sclerosis making use of mouthpiece ventilation (from Agrafiotis et al. [30], after permission).

ventilator until his lungs are maximally expanded. The maximum volume of air that can be held with a closed glottis is the patient's maximum insufflation capacity (MIC) [23]. The role of air-stacking is to preserve lung function by effecting lung volume recruitment and to avert chest wall strictures and contractures in patients with NMDs who experience a progressive decline in vital capacity (VC) [24, 25]. The difference MIC-VC depends directly on the integrity of glottic function and represents the amount of recruitable lung volume [24]. In a recent retrospective study of 151 patients with Duchenne muscular dystrophy (DMD), lung volume recruitment by air-stacking delayed the maximal VC decline by at least 5 years [26]. Other researchers have also reported a decrease in the rate of VC decline in patients with DMD [27] and a progressive increase in the MIC-VC difference, indicating a higher number of recruitable lung units [28]. In addition, lung expansion by air-stacking takes advantage of the increased respiratory system recoil pressure at high lung volumes to increase peak cough flow (PCF) and facilitate secretion clearance. In a group of 61 DMD patients, mean PCF increased from 137 to 236 L/min with the application of the air-stacking maneuver [29]. As an example, the application of air-stacking in a patient with amyotrophic lateral sclerosis (ALS) receiving MPV was associated with a MIC-VC difference of 0.4 L and an increase of PCF from 50 to 200 L/min [30]. Therefore, the use of MPV in combination with the air-stacking maneuver supports daytime ventilatory function and improves cough efficacy deferring tracheostomy.

GPB is another strategy commonly taught to MPV users. This technique is based on the use of the tongue to gulp consecutive boluses of air, while the glottis remains closed after each gulp to retain the inhaled air. By imitating the effects of a deep breath, GPB induces lung volume recruitment and improves cough efficacy. In addition, GPB provides ventilator independency for patients with limited off-ventilator time and can be used as a rescue strategy in case of an accidental mouthpiece disconnection or ventilator failure [5, 6, 31].

During the last years, the use of MPV has also expanded to patients with other chronic respiratory diseases such as chest wall diseases [32] as well as to acute exacerbations of chronic obstructive pulmonary disease (COPD) [33, 34]. Nevertheless, despite the increasing interest in MPV, its application is limited to few centers specializing in noninvasive respiratory management [35]. Many practitioners are unfamiliar with its use, and several authors still consider tracheostomy as the most effective and secure method of ventilation for patients with advanced diseases [1].

In the rest of the chapter, we will present the evidence supporting the application of MPV for the management of respiratory disease and address several practical issues related to its use.

2. Evidence

2.1. Mouthpiece ventilation for full-time ventilatory support in neuromuscular patients

The application of MPV ventilation to 75 post-polio survivors with chronic respiratory failure was reported by Bach et al. [5]. All patients were using MPV as a major part of their respiratory support, but some (31%) were also using body respirators and the majority (88%) required full-time ventilator assistance. On average MPV was used for 1028 patient-years (14.8 years per person) for a total mortality of 1 death per 60.5 patient-years. Several of these MPV users married and some also joined the workforce.

Toussaint et al. [8] reported on 42 patients with DMD treated with MPV. Before introduced to MPV, all patients had diurnal hypercapnia by the end of the day while being treated optimally with nocturnal nasal ventilation. Survival at 1, 3, 5 and 7 years was 88, 66, 58 and 51%, respectively. Importantly, the use of MPV was associated with stabilization of VC, despite a deterioration in respiratory muscle strength, while transcutaneous CO_2 values improved. Some patients also reported improvements in dyspnea, appetite and swallowing. No important accidents or complications were observed over the 7-year follow-up period. VC was also preserved in a small cohort of 12 DMD patients who were prescribed MPV, a fact attributed to the concurrent use of lung volume recruitment strategies [36].

MPV was also compared to tracheostomy ventilation (TV) in 42 patients with DMD [9]. All tracheostomized patients (n = 16) used cuffless tubes and speaking valves connected in line with the ventilator circuit. While TV was associated with a higher incidence of tracheal injuries, mucous hypersecretion and lung infections, MPV users had a slightly higher incidence of weight loss and need for enteral feeding. Causes of death did not roughly differ between the two groups, however one MPV user died as a result of loss of mouthpiece during wheelchair malfunction, while a TV patient died during an endoscopic procedure.

Bedard and McKim [10] reported retrospectively on the use of MPV in patients with ALS. Of 37 patients in total, 27 were considered to be successful MPV users (consistent use > 1 month). The majority of the successful patients had less severe bulbar symptoms and demonstrated recruitable lung volume with MIC > VC. Importantly, all successful users experienced improved dyspnea scores and normalization of CO_2 values. For this group of patients, FVC decreased as disease progressed, but MIC was relatively preserved and MIC-VC difference increased. The majority of them could effect a PCF > 180 L/min with lung volume recruitment throughout disease course. In addition, a PCF > 180 L/min at initiation of MPV in successful users was associated with significantly better mean survival (637 vs. 240 days).

In addition, Khirani et al. [37] obtained questionnaires on quality of life issues from 30 neuromuscular MPV users. The majority of the patients reported reductions in dyspnea (73%) and fatigue (93%), and some of them also improvements in the ease of speech (43%) and swallowing (27%).

Overall, the above evidence indicates that MPV may defer tracheostomy, improve or stabilize clinically relevant lung function variables and possibly improve quality of life and confer a survival benefit to neuromuscular patients. The application of MPV seems relatively safe, although the possibility of mouthpiece loss is not a negligible concern. In addition, the concurrent use of other noninvasive aids, e.g. mechanical insufflation-exsufflation devices, might bias the interpretation of these studies. From this point of view, it is worth noting that in the study by Toussaint et al. [8], mechanical insufflation-exsufflation was available for only 7% of the patients. Nevertheless, further prospective studies are warranted to explore the impact of MPV on the outcomes of neuromuscular patients.

2.2. Mouthpiece ventilation for "unweanable" ventilator-dependent neuromuscular patients

MPV, sometimes combined with mechanical insufflation-exsufflation, has been successfully employed as a noninvasive method of weaning or removal of artificial tubes for patients with acute or chronic ventilatory failure, the majority of which had various NMDs. Many of these patients continued using MPV for several years [5, 6, 38]. A recent study [7] evaluated a simplified protocol for the extubation of neuromuscular patients with no ventilator-free breathing time. All patients (n = 157) who were normocapnic on invasive mechanical ventilation could maintain an $SpO_2 > 95\%$ for 12 hours on room air and could reverse desaturations with the use of mechanical insufflation-exsufflation device were extubated to noninvasive nasal, oronasal or mouthpiece volume assisted-controlled ventilation. Intensive use of mechanical insufflation-exsufflation was provided after extubation. Patients using MPV could determine the amount of volume they required and, when possible, could wean themselves *after* extubation by taking gradually fewer breaths from the mouthpiece. This protocol effected extubation success (defined as discharge without reintubation) in 157 (98%) of the patients, of whom 46% remained full-time ventilator-dependent. Although this study does not provide specific data with respect to each interface, it does exemplify the usefulness of mouthpiece for providing full-time ventilatory support without the requirement of an invasive tube.

2.3. Mouthpiece ventilation in other chronic respiratory diseases

Nicolini et al. [32] recruited 18 mechanical ventilation-naive patients with severe kyphoscoliosis in a prospective 4-year study, which evaluated the impact of combined diurnal MPV and nocturnal MV on lung function, clinical outcomes and health-related quality of life. They observed significant improvements in spirometric indices, blood gases, static mouth pressures, ventilatory drive and polygraphic variables at 6 months. In addition, patients reported improvements in quality of life aspects as sleep, physical well-being, eating, leisure, self-confidence and mood. Mortality at the end of the study period was 22.2%. When compared to a historical group of kyphoscoliotic patients who received only nocturnal MV, survival was better for the combined group at 180, 360 and 720 days.

2.4. Mouthpiece ventilation in acute respiratory exacerbations

There is limited evidence on the effectiveness, safety and tolerance of MPV in the setting of acute respiratory failure. A randomized cross-over prospective physiologic study compared four different interfaces with various internal volumes including a mouthpiece with minimal internal volume in critically ill patients. No difference was noted in gas change and respiratory effort variables, but the mouthpiece was associated with more leaks and asynchronies and a significantly less comfort on a visual analogue scale [39]. In a cross-over study which compared short-term mouthpiece and face mask tolerance in a cohort of 27 intensive care unit (ICU) patients treated for acute respiratory failure, five patients were withdrawn due to poor tolerance of the mouthpiece. For the remaining subjects and their nurses, facemask was associated with a nonsignificant better comfort, but mouthpiece required a significantly higher nursing time. While oxygenation and blood gases significantly improved with both interfaces, only face masks were associated with a significantly lower respiratory rate [40].

Some of the above findings were challenged by more recent clinical studies. Glerant et al. [33] conducted a retrospective matched case-control study in which MPV was compared to nasal MV and standard medical care in 87 COPD patients admitted to a respiratory ICU due to acute hypercapnic exacerbation of mild severity (average pH 7.3). In both groups, assist-control or pressure support modes were used. MPV was applied for 20 minutes every hour during the day and at less frequent intervals during the night. All MPV patients used a nose clips and had to hold the mouthpiece firmly and keep their mouth closed to avoid leaks. This study observed a nonsignificant lower intubation rate for MPV as compared to MV users (7 vs. 14%) and similar improvements in blood gases although these changes occurred much later in the MPV group, a fact attributed to a longer learning period for these patients. Overall, the duration of NIV and ICU stay did not differ between these two groups.

The same question was revisited by a recent randomized controlled trial. Nicolini et al. [34] randomized 50 COPD patients presenting with acute exacerbation of mild-moderate severity (pH 7.25–7.30) to receive either nasal MV or MPV in the pressure support mode. No case of NIV failure was observed, and blood gas values showed similar trends while the duration of NIV and hospital stay did not differ between the two groups. Common complications included skin breakdown for the MV group and gastric distention for the MPV group. However, tolerance and device acceptability was better for the MPV group.

Criticism for both the abovementioned studies focused on the use of nasal masks in the setting of an acute exacerbation and the absence of long-term results. In addition, the study by Nicolini et al. [33] was underpowered to assess changes in blood gases, which was the primary outcome [41]. Pending the results of further investigations, MPV might be considered for COPD patients with a mild-moderate acute exacerbation who are intolerant of nasal or oronasal masks but retain a good level of consciousness and are not severely distressed in order to understand and apply this technique.

3. Practicalities in the application of mouthpiece ventilation

MPV is mainly indicated for neuromuscular patients with chronic ventilator failure when they develop daytime hypercapnia despite optimized nocturnal ventilatory support [8] or when they manifest deteriorating daytime breathlessness with increasing ventilator dependence [10]. MPV can be performed with (1) a home life-support ventilator, (2) a single or a double-limb circuit, (3) various types of mouthpieces, and (4) adjustable support arm or custom-made straps to mount the mouthpiece close to the head for patients with advanced motor disabilities (**Figure 2**). The presence of an exhalation valve in the circuit is not a prerequisite for the delivery of MPV; however, it might be necessary for switching to nocturnal MV for patients using non-vented circuits. The ideal candidate should be able to grab the mouthpiece with his lips and adequately rotate his neck [10]. MPV can be combined with MV during sleep or applied 24 hours per day using specifically designed interfaces [6, 31].

3.1. Patient education

Most of the patients considered for MPV have already been using MV for several years. Nevertheless, the experience of MPV is quite different and some patients may feel uncomfortable and express reluctance to continue. The application of MPV requires active participation

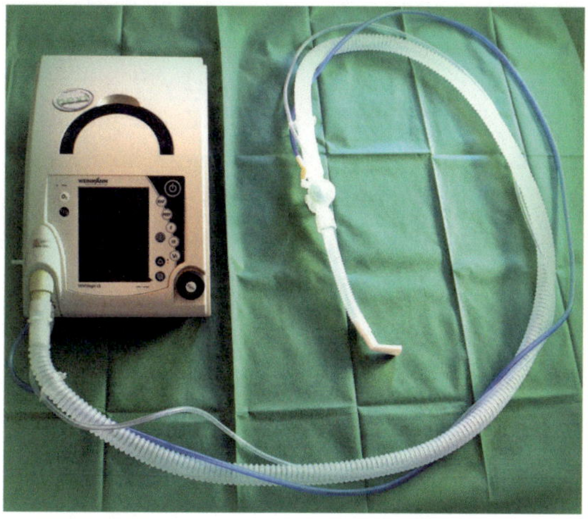

Figure 2. Setup for mouthpiece ventilation.

from the patient, increased nursing time and longer periods of training. We generally instruct patients to "sip" from the mouthpiece, in a manner similar to drinking a beverage using a straw (**Figure 1**). When this maneuver is applied, the soft palate moves posterocaudally sealing off the nasopharynx and minimizing nasal leaks. Importantly, the "sip" maneuver generates a higher negative pressure than maximum static inspiratory pressure, a fact that makes triggering easier for the frail neuromuscular patients [1].

3.2. Ventilator settings

The ventilator is usually set to the volume assisted-controlled mode with a Vt between 0.7 and 1.5 L, while PEEP (or EPAP) and backup rate are set to zero or to the lowest manufacturer-defined value. Recommendations on how to choose Vt and inspiratory time (Ti) are generally scarce [3]. If the patient is breathing comfortably while using MV, we begin with a similar Vt, albeit increased by 0.1–0.3 L to account for leaks and we commonly use a Ti at least as high as 1 s. Then we gradually increase Vt and/or Ti over several hours or days as much as tolerated. Many patients might have been using bilevel MV for many years before being introduced to volume-targeted MPV. While in bilevel ventilation, peak inspiratory flow is determined by the preset pressure, respiratory resistance and patient effort [42] in traditional volume-targeted ventilation inspiratory flow is ventilator-defined and is commonly delivered using a square waveform shape. Nevertheless, if the patient becomes severely breathless when switched to volume-targeted MPV, the use of a decelerating flow shape which delivers higher peak inspiratory flows at the start of the breath might be considered [43] . Generally, the patient should be able to define his own ventilatory pattern by determining the number of breaths and the quantity of leak [8]. Some experts would choose to use a pressure, rather than a flow-regulated, inspiratory trigger to avoid autotriggering [44]. However, despite the fact that in many new generation home ventilators only flow triggering is available, autotriggering with MPV seems to be less common than initially thought [37, 45]. Inspiratory trigger should be sensitive enough to reduce the work of breathing. However, since MPV users commonly fail to trigger the ventilator [45], a number of backup breaths could be set to ensure adequate ventilation and avert fatigue. On the other hand, machine-triggered breaths during patient disconnection from the mouthpiece might be a source of discomfort as a result of high flow on the user's face [45]. Nevertheless, in some newer generation ventilators, triggering can be simply effected by creating a small negative pressure at the mouthpiece ("kiss-trigger") [3, 37]. It must be noted that standard turbine ventilators are not designed to perform under conditions of rapidly changing load. A bench study which evaluated five different modern home ventilators observed significant swings in Vt when conditions of disconnection and reconnection were experimentally reproduced [46].

3.3. Alarms

One of the major problems in open-circuit systems is the prevention of "low pressure" and "apnea" alarm activation. As a general rule, these alarms should be switched off when possible or set to the lowest sensitive value allowed by the manufacturer. Several new generation home ventilators are more versatile in alarm customization with some even incorporating specifically designed software for MPV [37, 45]. Nevertheless, the use of high resistance mouthpieces together with smart combinations of Vt and Ti may create a sufficient back pressure which will prevent "low pressure" alarm activation, when the last cannot be switched off [37, 44]; practical recommendations for alarm customization for several home life-support ventilators have become recently available [45]. When 'apnea' alarming cannot be deactivated, a minimum of backup breaths should be set corresponding to the maximum allowed apnea time [44]. It should be noted, however, that at least in some types of ventilators, backup rate manipulation might also influence Ti, making alarm customization even more complicated [45].

3.4. Mouthpieces

There are a few types of mouthpieces available in the market nowadays, including angled 15 and 22 mm mouthpieces, straw-like as well as lip-sealing interfaces or orthodontic bite plates (**Figure 3**). The performance of these interfaces in the delivery of MPV has been assessed in a limited number of studies. Khirani et al. [37] compared three different angled mouthpiece configurations, a large mouthpiece (22 mm) and a small mouthpiece (15 mm) with and without a filter in a bench study which validated six different types of life-support home ventilators. The resistance was higher with the 15 mm mouthpiece with a filter, and this configuration was also

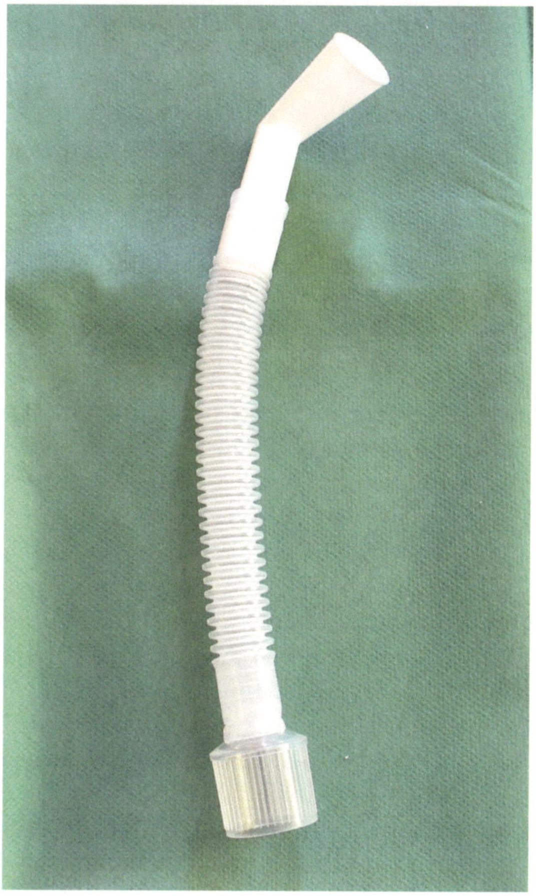

Figure 3. A 15 mm mouthpiece.

associated with a lower incidence of "low pressure" alarm activation. In another bench study, Ogna et al. [47] used four different home ventilators to compare the mechanical properties of various mouthpieces including a newly designed one. With respect to the most commonly used interfaces, respiratory resistance was lower with the 15 mm rigid-angled mouthpiece and higher with the straw mouthpiece. In volume-targeted modes with a Vt set to 1 L, both interfaces performed equally well across the different ventilators in delivering a volume close to the predetermined, while in pressure-targeted modes the effective pressure with the straw mouthpiece was slighter lower as a result of the increased resistance. The clinical implications of these findings remain unclear. For the time being, the choice of the interface should be tailored to the individual needs of each patient. An angled 15 mm mouthpiece seems to be a rational choice because its configuration increases resistance to the airflow preventing the activation of the "low pressure" alarm and in addition it is easier for the patient to grab [1]. If "low pressure" alarming persists, the addition of a filter to the circuit might be a simple and practical solution to the problem [37]. In addition, MPV can also be delivered during sleep with the use of specifically designed orthodontic bite plates or lip-sealing retention systems with attached Velcro straps to avoid disconnection. The use of these interfaces might cause desaturation, fragmented sleep and repeated arousals in a minority of the patients due to nasal leakage. Nasal pledges or clips can be applied to patients with significant nasal leaks [31].

3.5. Speaking and deglutition

Speaking is commonly problematic in patients with advanced respiratory disease as it requires higher than tidal inspiratory volumes and may slow the breathing rate causing breathlessness and fatigue [48]. If a patient on MPV needs to speak, he must take a large breath from the mouthpiece and then speak while expiration is driven by the expiratory muscles and the respiratory system recoil pressure. Nevertheless, speaking with the use of the mouthpiece might be associated with longer pauses (in order to breath in) and difficulties in choosing the right strategy for mouthpiece positioning and use [48].

Breathing and swallowing are normally competitive procedures and their coordination is disrupted in respiratory disease with respiration taking precedence over swallowing. Swallowing in neuromuscular patients is characterized by piecemeal deglutition, increased time to swallow a bolus and an increased number of swallows during inspiration. The institution of positive pressure ventilation stabilizes breathing and improves swallowing performance [49]. The practice of MPV should theoretically contribute to the restoration of swallowing and breathing coordination as users have to alternate between taking deep breaths from the mouthpiece and swallowing. In addition, MPV should also maintain the supraglottic pressure required for effective swallowing, while the high inspired volumes improve cough efficacy providing protection against aspiration [48]. Nevertheless, as disease progresses and ventilator-free time is reduced, less time is available for swallowing, while the presence of food in the mouth and in the pharynx does not allow patients to breath in safely. To deal with this problem, some patients use the ventilator to perform air-stacking in order to increase lung volume and afford longer periods of apnea without breathlessness [9]. Although weight loss and feeding problems in MPV users have been reported [9], it is not clear whether these should be attributed to the interface *per se* or to disease progression and increasing breathlessness.

It should be noted that a disconnection from the mouthpiece for eating and speaking might compromise effective gas exchange. In a small study including eight MPV users who were monitored with polygraghy during daily activities, most of the patients could speak and eat without ventilator assistance; however, prolonged disconnections (>3 min) (e.g. during meals) were associated with significant drops in SpO_2 and increases in transcutaneous PCO_2 [50].

3.6. Complications

A few complications associated with MPV have been so far reported, of which mouthpiece loss is the most important [9]. This complication can be avoided if the mouthpiece's position is secured using specifically designed support arms or customary-made straps. Fixation of the mouthpiece on the shoulders allows the interface to follow the patient's movements [8]. In addition, MPV users could be taught the technique of GPB to maintain ventilator independency in case of accidental mouthpiece loss [6, 31]. Other complications include salivation, aerophagia, abdominal distention and orthodontic problems [1, 2, 6, 51]. There are no available data on the management of excessive salivation in mouthpiece users. For more severe cases the administration of an anticholinergic agent such as amitriptyline might be considered [9, 52]. Aerophagia and abdominal distention are common complications of noninvasive ventilatory support and have been associated with respiratory distress and ventilator dependence [51]. For patients with gastrostomies, unclamping the gastric tube to "burp out" the air is a quick method to effect symptom relief. Sometimes a nasogastric or a rectal rube (for patients with colonic distention) might also be helpful [51]. For patients with persistent symptoms switching to pressure-targeted ventilation could be an option, although this mode is not suitable for the application of lung volume recruitment and air-stacking maneuvers. If the patient is maintained on a volume-targeted mode, setting a lower pressure limit to effect secondary pressure cycling is an alternative option. Vomiting and aspiration as a result of gastric distention as well as pneumothorax have been so far theoretical concerns, but they represent potentially life-threatening events [4, 53]. Orthodontic complications are not uncommon in long-term users; however, they pose mostly an esthetic rather than a functional concern and specifically designed orthodontic interfaces have become available in the market [6, 31, 53]. Patients on MPV and full-time ventilator dependence can safely undergo dental procedures using nasal interfaces as long as oxygen saturation is monitored and oxygen or sedatives are avoided [54].

4. Conclusion

MPV is a "re-discovered" method of noninvasive ventilation that can be used to provide full-time ventilatory support, recruit lung volume, improve cough efficacy, defer tracheostomy and possibly improve survival and quality of life in neuromuscular patients. MPV might also be beneficial for patients with other chronic respiratory diseases or in acute COPD hypercapnic exacerbation. The successful application of MPV requires careful selection of patient, interface, ventilator and alarm settings, increased nursing time and comprehensive patient training.

Conflict of interest

None for all authors.

Funding

This work was supported by the Hellenic Society of Respiratory and Occupational Lung Diseases

Author details

Michalis Agrafiotis*, Konstantina Nikolaou, Dimitra Siopi and Diamantis Chloros

*Address all correspondence to: m.agrafiotis@gmail.com

Department of Pulmonary Medicine, Respiratory Neuromuscular Outpatient Clinic, "Georgios Papanikolaou" General Hospital of Thessaloniki, Exohi, Greece

References

[1] Pinto T, Chatwin M, Banfi P, Winck JC, Nicolini A. Mouthpiece ventilation and complementary techniques in patients with neuromuscular disease: A brief clinical review and update. Chronic Respiratory Disease. May 2017;**14**(2):187-193

[2] Benditt JO. Full-time noninvasive ventilation: possible and desirable. Respiratory Care. Sep 2006;**51**(9):1005-1012

[3] Garuti G, Nicolini A, Grecchi B, Lusuardi M, Winck JC, Bach JR. Open circuit mouthpiece ventilation: Concise clinical review. Revista Portuguesa de Pneumologia. Jul–Aug 2014;**20**(4): 211-218

[4] Bach JR, Alba AS, Bohatiuk G, Saporito L, Lee M. Mouth intermittent positive pressure ventilation in the management of postpolio respiratory insufficiency. Chest. Jun 1987;**91**(6): 859-864

[5] Bach JR, Alba AS. Noninvasive options for ventilatory support of the traumatic high level quadriplegic patient. Chest. Sep 1990;**98**(3):613-619

[6] Bach JR, Alba AS, Saporito LR. Intermittent positive pressure ventilation via the mouth as an alternative to tracheostomy for 257 ventilator users. Chest. Jan 1993;**103**(1):174-182

[7] Bach JR, Gonçalves MR, Hamdani I, Winck JC. Extubation of patients with neuromuscular weakness: A new management paradigm. Chest. May 2010;**137**(5):1033-1039

[8] Toussaint M, Steens M, Wasteels G, Soudon P. Diurnal ventilation via mouthpiece: Survival in end-stage Duchenne patients. The European Respiratory Journal. Sep 2006;**28**(3):549-555

[9] Soudon P, Steens M, Toussaint M. A comparison of invasive versus noninvasive full-time mechanical ventilation in Duchenne muscular dystrophy. Chronic Respiratory Disease. 2008;**5**(2):87-93

[10] Bédard ME, McKim DA. Daytime mouthpiece for continuous noninvasive ventilation in individuals with amyotrophic lateral sclerosis. Respiratory Care. Oct 2016;**61**(10): 1341-1348

[11] Benditt JO. The neuromuscular respiratory system: Physiology, pathophysiology, and a respiratory care approach to patients. Respiratory Care. Aug 2006;**51**(8):829-837

[12] Benditt JO, Boitano LJ. Pulmonary issues in patients with chronicneuromuscular disease. American Journal of Respiratory and Critical Care Medicine. May 15, 2013;**187**(10):1046-1055

[13] Ragette R, Mellies U, Schwake C, Voit T, Teschler H. Patterns and predictors of sleep disordered breathing in primary myopathies. Thorax. Aug 2002;**57**(8):724-728

[14] Simonds AK, Muntoni F, Heather S, Fielding S. Impact of nasal ventilation on survival in hypercapnic Duchenne muscular dystrophy. Thorax. Nov 1998;**53**(11):949-952

[15] Jeppesen J, Green A, Steffensen BF, Rahbek J. The Duchenne muscular dystrophy population in Denmark, 1977-2001: Prevalence, incidence and survival in relation to the introduction of ventilator use. Neuromuscular Disorders. Dec 2003;**13**(10):804-812

[16] Ward S, Chatwin M, Heather S, Simonds AK. Randomised controlled trial of non-invasive ventilation (NIV) for nocturnal hypoventilation in neuromuscular and chest wall disease patients with daytime normocapnia. Thorax. Dec 2005;**60**(12):1019-1024

[17] Bourke SC, Tomlinson M, Williams TL, Bullock RE, Shaw PJ, Gibson GJ. Effects of non-invasive ventilation on survival and quality of life in patients with amyotrophic lateral sclerosis: A randomised controlled trial. Lancet Neurology. Feb 2006;**5**(2):140-147

[18] Vrijsen B, Buyse B, Belge C, Robberecht W, Van Damme P, Decramer M, Testelmans D. Noninvasive ventilation improves sleep in amyotrophic lateral sclerosis: A prospective polysomnographic study. Journal of Clinical Sleep Medicine. Apr 15, 2015;**11**(5):559-566

[19] Boentert M, Brenscheidt I, Glatz C, Young P. Effects of non-invasive ventilation on objective sleep and nocturnal respiration in patients with amyotrophic lateral sclerosis. Journal of Neurology. Sep 2015;**262**(9):2073-2082

[20] King AC. Long-term home mechanical ventilation in the United States. Respiratory Care. Jun 2012;**57**(6):921-930

[21] Lloyd-Owen SJ, Donaldson GC, Ambrosino N, Escarabill J, Farre R, Fauroux B, Robert D, Schoenhofer B, Simonds AK, Wedzicha JA. Patterns of home mechanical ventilation use in Europe: Results from the Eurovent survey. The European Respiratory Journal. Jun 2005;**25**(6):1025-1031

[22] Bach JRA. Comparison of long-term ventilatory support alternatives from the perspective of the patient and care giver. Chest. Dec 1993;**104**(6):1702-1706

[23] Kang SW, Bach JR. Maximum insufflation capacity. Chest. 2000 Jul;**118**(1):61-65

[24] Ishikawa Y, Bach JR. Physical medicine respiratory muscle aids to avert respiratory complications of pediatric chest wall and vertebral deformity and muscle dysfunction. European Journal of Physical and Rehabilitation Medicine. 2010 Dec;**46**(4):581-597

[25] Molgat-Seon Y, Hannan LM, Dominelli PB, Peters CM, Fougere RJ, McKim DA, Sheel AW, Road JD. Lung volume recruitment acutely increases respiratory system compliance in individuals with severe respiratory muscle weakness. ERJ Open Research. Mar 14, 2017;**3**(1):00135-2016

[26] Chiou M, Bach JR, Jethani L, Gallagher MF. Active lung volume recruitment to preserve vital capacity in Duchenne muscular dystrophy. Journal of Rehabilitation Medicine. Jan 19, 2017;**49**(1):49-53

[27] Katz SL, Barrowman N, Monsour A, Su S, Hoey L, McKim D. Long-term effects of lung volume recruitment on maximal inspiratory capacity and vital capacity in Duchenne muscular dystrophy. Annals of the American Thoracic Society. Feb 2016;**13**(2):217-222

[28] Bach JR, Mahajan K, Lipa B, Saporito L, Goncalves M, Komaroff E. Lung insufflation capacity in neuromuscular disease. American Journal of Physical Medicine & Rehabilitation. Sep 2008;**87**(9):720-725

[29] Ishikawa Y, Bach JR, Komaroff E, Miura T, Jackson-Parekh R. Cough augmentation in Duchenne muscular dystrophy. American Journal of Physical Medicine & Rehabilitation. Sep 2008;**87**(9):726-730

[30] Agrafiotis M, Renessis V, Kousta A, Athanassiadou A, Tryfon S, Chloros D. Noninvasive ventilation via a mouthpiece in a patient with amyotrophic lateral sclerosis. Pneumon. Jan–Mar 2017;**30**(1) (in press)

[31] Bach JR. Continuous noninvasive ventilation for patients with neuromuscular disease and spinal cord injury. Seminars in Respiratory and Critical Care Medicine. Jun 2002;**23**(3): 283-292

[32] Nicolini A, Barlascini C, Piroddi IM, Garuti G, Banfi PI. Effectiveness and safety of mouthpiece ventilation and nocturnal non-invasive ventilation in patients with kyphoscoliosis: Short and long-term outcomes after an episode of acute respiratory failure. Revista Portuguesa de Pneumologia (2006). Mar–Apr 2016;**22**(2):75-81

[33] Glerant JC, Rose D, Oltean V, Dayen C, Mayeux I, Jounieaux V. Noninvasive ventilation using a mouthpiece in patients with chronic obstructive pulmonary disease and acute respiratory failure. Respiration. 2007;**74**(6):632-639

[34] Nicolini A, Santo M, Ferrari-Bravo M, Barlascini C. Open-mouthpiece ventilation versus nasal mask ventilation in subjects with COPD exacerbation and mild to moderate acidosis: A randomized trial. Respiratory Care. Dec 2014;**59**(12):1825-1831

[35] Bach JR, Gonçalves MR, Hon A, Ishikawa Y, De Vito EL, Prado F, Dominguez ME. Changing trends in the management of end-stage neuromuscular respiratory muscle failure: Recommendations of an international consensus. American Journal of Physical Medicine & Rehabilitation. Mar 2013;**92**(3):267-277

[36] McKim DA, Griller N, LeBlanc C, Woolnough A, King J. Twenty-four hour noninvasive ventilation in Duchenne muscular dystrophy: A safe alternative to tracheostomy. Canadian Respiratory Journal. Jan–Feb 2013;**20**(1):e5-e9

[37] Khirani S, Ramirez A, Delord V, Leroux K, Lofaso F, Hautot S, Toussaint M, Orlikowski D, Louis B, Fauroux B. Evaluation of ventilators for mouthpiece ventilation in neuromuscular disease. Respiratory Care. Sep 2014;**59**(9):1329-1337

[38] Bach JR, Saporito LR. Criteria for extubation and tracheostomy tube removal for patients with ventilatory failure. A different approach to weaning. Chest. Dec 1996;**110**(6):1566-1571

[39] Fraticelli AT, Lellouche F, L'her E, Taillé S, Mancebo J, Brochard L. Physiological effects of different interfaces during noninvasive ventilation for acute respiratory failure. Critical Care Medicine. Mar 2009;**37**(3):939-945

[40] Schneider E, Dualé C, Vaille JL, Ouchchane L, Gillart T, Guélon D, Schoeffler P. Comparison of tolerance of facemask vs. mouthpiece for non-invasive ventilation. Anaesthesia. Jan 2006;**61**(1):20-23

[41] Carlucci A, Gregoretti C. Mouthpiece ventilation: Just a home-care support? Respiratory Care. Dec 2014;**59**(12):1951-1953

[42] Hess DR. Ventilator waveforms and the physiology of pressure support ventilation. Respiratory Care. Feb 2005;**50**(2):166-186

[43] Agrafiotis M, Kotsifou E, Renessis V, Athanassiadou A, Kousta A, Chloros D. Decelerating flow shape for volume-targeted mouthpiece ventilation. The Clinical Respiratory Journal. (in press)

[44] Boitano LJ, Benditt JO. An evaluation of home volume ventilators that support open-circuit mouthpiece ventilation. Respiratory Care. Nov 2005;**50**(11):1457-1461

[45] Carlucci A, Mattei A, Rossi V, Paracchini E, Raineri SM, Gregoretti C. Ventilator settings to avoid nuisance alarms during mouthpiece ventilation. Respiratory Care. Apr 2016;**61**(4): 462-467

[46] Ogna A, Prigent H, Falaize L, Leroux K, Santos D, Vaugier I, Orlikowski D, Lofaso F. Accuracy of tidal volume delivered by home mechanical ventilation during mouthpiece ventilation: A bench evaluation. Chronic Respiratory Disease. May 3, 2016. pii: 1479972316647177

[47] Ogna A, Prigent H, Falaize L, Leroux K, Santos D, Vaugier I, Orlikowski D, Lofaso F. Bench evaluation of commercially available and newly developed interfaces for mouthpiece ventilation. The Clinical Respiratory Journal. Dec 27, 2016 (in press)

[48] Britton D, Benditt JO, Hoit JD. Beyond tracheostomy: Noninvasive ventilation and potential positive implications for speaking and swallowing. Seminars in Speech and Language. Aug 2016;**37**(3):173-184

[49] Terzi N, Orlikowski D, Prigent H, Denise P, Normand H, Lofaso F. Noninvasive monitoring of breathing and swallowing interaction. In: Mark Schwartz EMG Methods for Evaluating Muscle and Nerve Function. In-tech; 2012. ISBN: 978-953-307-793-2. Available from: http://www.intechopen.com/books/emgmethods-or-evaluating-muscle-and-nerve-function/noninvasive-monitoring-of-breathing-and-swallowinginteraction

[50] Nardi J, Leroux K, Orlikowski D, Prigent H, Lofaso F. Home monitoring of daytime mouthpiece ventilation effectiveness in patients with neuromuscular disease. Chronic Respiratory Disease. Feb 2016;**13**(1):67-74

[51] Bach JR, Mehta AD. Respiratory muscle aids to avert respiratory failure and tracheostomy: A new patient management paradigm. Journal of Neurorestoratology. 2014;**2**:25-35

[52] Banfi P, Ticozzi N, Lax A, Guidugli GA, Nicolini A, Silani V. A review of options for treating sialorrhea in amyotrophic lateral sclerosis. Respiratory Care. Mar 2015;**60**(3):446-454

[53] Nava S, Navalesi P, Gregoretti C. Interfaces and humidification for noninvasive mechanical ventilation. Respiratory Care. Jan 2009;**54**(1):71-84

[54] Tran J, Bach JR, Gonçalves MR. Alternatives to mouthpiece noninvasive ventilatory support to permit dental care. American Journal of Physical Medicine & Rehabilitation. Feb 2014;**93**(2):182-185